TWO'S COMPANY

By the same authors:
Praying Together

Two's Company

Testament of childlessness

MIKE & KATEY MORRIS

KINGSWAY PUBLICATIONS
EASTBOURNE

Unless otherwise indicated, biblical quotations are from
the Holy Bible: New International Version, copyright ©
International Bible Society 1973, 1978, 1984.
The poem *Jill and Ben* is copyright © Stewart Henderson
1987.

Front cover photo: The Image Bank

British Library Cataloguing in Publication Data

    Morris, Mike
        Two's company: testament of
        childlessness
        1. Childlessness
        I. Title II. Morris, Katey
        362.8 HQ755.8

        ISBN 0-86065-583-0

Printed in Great Britain for
KINGSWAY PUBLICATIONS LTD
Lottbridge Drove, Eastbourne, E. Sussex BN23 6NT by
Richard Clay Ltd, Bungay, Suffolk.
Typeset by CST, Eastbourne, E. Sussex.

To parentless children everywhere

Acknowledgements

Grateful thanks to Carolyn 'fingers' Abbot who 'whizzed' through the manuscript translating hieroglyphics into typed copy, and to her patient husband John and delightful daughter Natalie.

To Stewart and Carol Henderson (not forgetting Maisie May!) for much encouragement, valued humour and sensitive insights. How delightful acquaintances can become friends!

To Lyndon and Celia Bowring for their constructive comments concerning presentation, and a most generous foreword.

And last, but not least, to the esteemed and learned Mr Christopher Catherwood: editor, adviser, friend. Who could ask for more than an enterprising editor to interpret the vagaries of his writers so precisely?

Thank you all so very much!

Preface

Jill and Ben

Is it her or is it him?
Two bruised, barren cherubim
thinking, 'Is this sacred whim
that out of her comes no more him?'

Is it him or is it her?
Shuffling in a doctor's chair,
screaming heart—but tidy hair
In his seed there's no more her

And this is what the man should do
To tame and impregnate his Shrew
amidst much laddish ballyhoo,
and this is what some men can't do

Once a womb, but now a dam
Outside Tesco's, change of plan—
steal a baby from a pram
then blame it on Fate's random ban

So is it him or is it her
whose organs seem beyond repair
whilst listening to the world's blank jeer
'Now is it him or is it her?'

Stewart Henderson

Foreword

Childlessness is as old as Abraham and Sarah, if not older! However, only in recent years, with the growing disintegration of family and community life, and the ensuing greater need for the security of family life, has the pain of childlessness become particularly unbearable for some.

Mike and Katey Morris are good friends of ours and we would have been glad to write this foreword for that reason; but because we were classified childless for five years in the early years of our marriage, we do have some feeling and understanding about the subject. God has since blessed us with two lovely children of our own, but this has not erased the memories of heartache and disappointment, the threat to our masculinity and femininity respectively, and the pain of thoughtless questions and comments.

Modern technology and medicine have encouraged us to believe that all things are possible for the childless couple. This, together with society's growing demands for life—when, where and how we wish—has blurred the truth that ultimately life is a supreme gift of God's grace. The question that people often ask is, 'How should we view some of the modern methods of helping couples to have a child of their own?' and we are in serious danger of demanding the experience and gift of a child, when God is maybe saying 'no!' The issue of childlessness raises all manner of questions—which Mike and Katey address honestly and helpfully.

This book will serve as a reminder to those who were childless, and are now parents; a challenge to those who are still without children and longing for parenthood, and a salutary reminder to couples who have not been faced with this problem. It is important for us all to be willing to enter into the lonely and painful experience of our friends and family in order for us to be to them all that we could be, and *Two's Company* will help us to achieve this goal.

Lyndon and Celia Bowring

Introduction

The camera pans around the hospital room filled with an assortment of multi-coloured flowers and congratulatory cards. Finally it zooms in to concentrate upon a smiling couple, complete with a babe in arms. As our TV screens provide an eloquent picture story, the words of the reporter convey a message about the wonders of modern science and its ability to free yet one more couple from the despair of childlessness. Interviewed, the couple speak of their own obvious joy, and why not? Then skilfully the interviewer draws them towards defining childlessness in terms reminiscent of a life sentence on some isolated gulag. An emotive case is immediately established for the application of the skill and finance of the medical sciences to concentrate on releasing as many from the blight of infertility as possible.

In these days of In Vitro Fertilization (IVF),

test-tube babies, surrogacy, Warnock and others, we are all aware of the wonders of modern medicine with regard to creating children. However, we are probably totally uninformed or ill-informed when it comes to infertility as such.

We discover that there is a major group of disadvantaged people within our society who can be described in this way. Ruthlessly discriminated against by nature, or so it would appear, couples unable to produce children find themselves excluded from the heart of much of the life in our family-based society. What is more, many have no one to whom they can turn for comfort and support. This often leaves a deep-seated feeling of isolation and rejection. Hence this book on infertility!

Mike and I have wrestled and wept, shouted and screamed during our journey from fearing we might face difficulties conceiving children to discovering the harsh reality that we have in fact less than a 1% chance of fertilization and pregnancy. It was not until we entered upon this journey that we discovered that our experience was shared by one in seven couples. It wasn't until we faced the issue personally that we realized how isolating an experience it can be and how little practical understanding there was from those with families. We write therefore as disadvantaged people to other disadvantaged people —those who share a common experience of infertility. We also write for all those who have and enjoy children, that they might learn second hand something of the world of the childless, enabling them to make creative strides towards them. One thing is clear: painful though infertility can be, it must never be allowed to rob us of friendships and relationships with others—or the pain becomes as persistent as the water from an ever-dripping tap; eventually it wears us away completely and, as well as the power to produce children, we yield the power to live life at all.

Many are the childless couples we have spoken with and, our own experience included, one of the most difficult pressures to adjust to is the fact that we live in an instant age. It was Access, the credit-card company, who first coined the phrase: 'Access takes the waiting out of wanting.' The campaign was an all time winner (we know the bankrupts to prove it!). All of us are educated to want the material maximum with minimum effort or delay. Unfortunately, what Access could do for the immediacy of ownership, they were unable to do for the real cost involved. Hence the sorry sight of millions of folk heavily in debt, each with a heart-rending tale to tell. Their fate? To pay a far higher price in real terms for goods they were not able to resist purchasing!

The effect of such advertising campaigns, reflecting the underlying expectation of society that we enjoy what amounts to a divine right to receive whatever we request, is not lost on the infertile. A child is their natural expectation. When children do not appear, then a major crisis of confidence and personal esteem descends. This is heightened against the back-drop of such divine-right mentality. This directs the couple's attention away from focusing on such questions as how to handle the aching in the waiting. This is a fundamental issue for any infertile couple. This is true of our journey and the book seeks to present honestly and helpfully the details of that journey and our reactions throughout. In writing this book, Mike and I have struggled faithfully to represent what each of us felt at various stages along our journey. We both decided, for reasons of style, that the final account should be written by my pen and trust this will prove to the reader's benefit.

As we look back over seven years of childlessness, we can see where we have grown as individuals; where we have met with and appreciated God along the way; where we have grown closer to one another. As you begin reading this journal, for such it is, being a record of our adventures thus far, expect the pain to be addressed and the hurt to be healed. If you are not childless expect to grow in understanding the plight of the childless and be a friend to them wherever they may be.

Chapter One

DIARY

The bell rang; my heart leapt. I raised my voice to give an impression of control but my words were lost amidst the scraping of chairs, slamming of desks and shrieks of delight. Within five minutes, my classroom was empty save for myself and the well-worn furniture—I felt pretty well worn myself; fine companion for the furniture!

As I gathered my gear together, my mind looked forward. It was Friday afternoon; it was May; it was the start of half-term! What joy; what delight coursed through my mortal frame.

Spring! Always an evocative time of year. Bright mornings, clear skies and the air heavy with the scent of distant childhood memories. What was it about spring which encouraged the mind to wander uninstructed down the long pathways of idle day-dreams?

A cheery 'Goodbye!' brought me back down to earth with a bump. I grunted some incomprehensible felicitation in response and immediately thought of Janet, now leaving for a half-term break with husband James and two young children. My heart burned warm at the thought of children; children of my own.

Lost in my reverie, I hardly noticed the car journey until I was dropped home. I waved off my commuting comrades and gladly entered the house, looking forward to a cup of tea and, eventually, Mike's return.

COMMENTARY

Mike and I had met while I was training to be a teacher in Oxford. Having completed my course, we moved to Wolverhampton in the West Midlands. Here I secured a teaching post immediately and Mike began working for British Youth for Christ on a voluntary basis whilst exploring possible career opportunities. Wolverhampton was a new experience for us both. We had grown up in the south-east of England, yet quickly fell in love with our new abode. Our house was 'user friendly' and we made some good friends. In fact, these were to prove our happiest years until finally settling in Chichester—but we had no inkling of this at the time.

School was another matter altogether! It was a split-site, multi-racial, inner-city comprehensive in the heart of an educational priority area. My eyes were opened in a way I would never have imagined and my heart went out to the children, many from the most desperate of backgrounds. Here was I, product of a fine girls public school, brought up in a comfortable, middle-class home, having to educate youngsters facing anything from desertion to incest! It was a challenge but one I enjoyed, in spite of the fact that it drew every ounce of energy from me. Mike proved a great support (after minimal training, I might add!), the more so through his work of meeting similar youngsters in the very different environment of youth evangelism.

DIARY

Half-term—sanity—sighs of relief: aaaaaaah! On reflection, our sanity was preserved by another couple and their family. It was amazing to see how Mike was able to relax and play with their kids—donkey rides, playhouses, endless stories; Mike excelled and revelled in them all. As I watched him, I promised myself that I would give him children of his own—he was apparently the perfect father (surely I'm not blinded by bias). I could imagine his excitement the day I proudly announced that I was pregnant. Goose-pimples just thinking about it. How wonderful is the imagination.

Two years teaching completed and sensing that I had done well in my chosen profession, my heart was stirring with desire for a child. I was twenty-five and had worked out that I wanted to have my children by the time I was thirty. Mike had always encouraged me to fulfil the 'teaching bug' as he termed it and once I knew it was out of my system, to consider starting a family. It had been good to have two years of marriage but now I felt that our home and marriage would be enriched with a new arrival. Mike has some time off over half-term and we must talk through the whole issue and make plans for the next stage of our lives. A resolution for half-term—how forthright! Today I'm a leader taking decisions. Watch out world!

Thinking about it, I could almost see those laughter lines on Mike's face radiating joy and happiness as I told him I wanted to start a family. With that thought reverberating around my mind, I drifted off to sleep, convinced that life is good . . . waking with a start, I realized that the key was turning in the front door. Consciousness reasserted itself as the door slammed, a characteristic of Mike's entrances. Mike home expecting food and nothing thought of, let alone prepared.

'Let's go out to eat and celebrate half-term in style.'

Casual suggestion accepted; phew! Credibility maintained yet again. What innovation. I really must be that leader!

May 1980 Funny thing, talking of starting a family seems fairly clinical and unemotional. Odd to think one determines when a new life begins:

'OK kid, now's your moment!'

Hey presto—bawling bundle of baby. Is this an insight into creation? We needs must project ahead and work out when it would be best to get pregnant and how much time I had to give with regard to my notice. Would school cope without me? Oh, the need to be needed! And yet motherhood beckoned and who could need me more than a vulnerable infant and a ham-fisted father!

Mike was travelling a fair bit and had always been insistent that once we had children, he would actively limit the number of miles he covered each year and the time he was away from home. There are issues for him to face and arrive at a practical solution. No doubt, content for a long evening discussion here.

COMMENTARY

Little did we think that our plans once made would meet with difficulties—but we were actually embarking on an adventure which would cause us to dig deeper into ourselves and cause our Christian convictions to be tested beyond anything we could have imagined.

About three months before our wedding, I had started taking the Pill. I found out about other forms of contraception but it seemed to be the obvious choice. It was reliable and convenient. Furthermore, at that time (1978) its disadvantages were not sufficient to cause me to reject it as I might were I starting today. I had been on the Pill before, as a teenager. I had been troubled by severe period pain. It was quite normal to take 'hormones', as the doctors called the Pill, to ease dysmenorrhoea and I had taken it for about two years. I suffered no side effects and therefore didn't hesitate to ask for it when I went for family-planning advice.

DIARY

July 1979 Smear tests!! Yuk: cold, metallic, medical instrument invading a very personal anatomical area. Men do not know the half of it! However, I always take such tests seriously and was grateful for the reassurance they gave. Today was the day for one such regular test—I took the opportunity to raise the issue of wanting to start a family.

My lady doctor was most sympathetic and understanding. She took time to explain that in her opinion it was advisable to have a three-month gap between coming off the Pill and seeking to conceive. This allowed all the chemical effects of the Pill to clear my body. As I left the surgery, she wished me luck!

Walking home, I felt both excited at the prospect of having a baby and also frustrated at having to wait three whole months! How can I perceive of eternity when three months seems such an unimaginably long period of time? Funny, I guess I'm just a 'NOW' person—always was and so shall continue to be! My sense of delayed gratification is somewhat impoverished; to consider God, heaven, eternity . . . well, I'd best leave it to the theologians. Stopped brain mid-thought and focused on the one concept I could grasp: 'I want a baby—NOW!'

It was July, so all systems would be go as from October. Mmmmm! A summer baby; that appealed. Indeed, it was a very welcome thought.

When does one begin searching through the name books? Come to that, where can I borrow some from? Would the library prove helpful? I need advice from experienced mothers.

COMMENTARY

Those three months did pass—slowly! But we had the added excitement of a move, owing to changes in Mike's job situation. All the arrangements for selling and buying consumed our energies for which I was grateful. In fact, having grown up in just the one house, moving came as something of a shock. It was amazing how the transit load of belongings we had originally transported to Wolverhampton following our student days had grown into a removal lorry load. The fruit of materialism.

In looking at houses, we were conscious of finding one suitable for a new-born babe. The end of November saw us packed and away, with the phrase 'New house, new baby' to the forefront of our minds. We had told no one of our plans, but a young couple in their mid-twenties with two years of marriage behind them are often expected to start 'producing'. Both subtle and not so subtle comments were made at times in our presence; we fended them all off valiantly if not a little too vigorously.

Moving is exhausting, time consuming and emotionally disturbing. With the move behind us, a new area and home to explore, I looked forward to a new addition to the family.

I had obviously resigned from my teaching job and I was in no rush to secure another. After all, I gave myself until the new year to 'settle down' and it hardly seemed worth taking a job only to have to resign upon becoming pregnant. I had reached the interview stage of one job and when I didn't get it, I saw it as the Lord planning my imminent pregnancy! What other reason could there be for preventing so prolific a talent from re-entering the teaching profession! Throughout this time, we would idly chat about babies whilst casting novices' eyes over Mothercare catalogues—yes, even Mike.

Diary

Christmas Day 1979 Christmas came and went. Blink and you miss it. All that energy, excitement and enthusiasm, only to sense at the end of it all you've missed something, somewhere, somehow. Such raw emotion channelling all energy towards a single day in the calendar cannot be healthy. No wonder people over-eat, drink in excess and engage in hollow hilarity so fervently. Everyone vainly trying to make the connection between intense, up-market pre-Christmas anticipation and the day itself.

Arrived back from friends early Christmas morning. Good time; good friends; God bless 'em.

Arose late; exchanged presents—a book on caring for house-plants from Mike. He went into raptures over my thoughtful and imaginative gift, exotically wrapped and endearingly ripped open by his eager, investigative hands. The gift? One pair of sparkling, new bicycle clips! Money in short supply but the occasion suitably marked.

Christmas Day together. Sad in a way; few goodies which one associates with the festive season, owing to financial constraints. We consoled each other by discussing Christmas a year hence when we would have a baby to entertain and be entertained by.

Night fell—TV movie gave way to TV movie and eventually bed beckoned. Not a Christmas to be recorded in 'memorable moments I have known and loved'; by New Year it will all be a fast-fading moment if not a figment of my diseased imagination.

Boxing Day The parents tour. Traditions from childhood re-enacted and prove very reassuring. Evident parental desire for grandchildren—very kindly and graciously communicated. Day ends with Mike standing to attention, saluting and pledging to do his duty for Queen and Country. I am far too well 'brung' up to say more . . . we shall move on!

COMMENTARY

Mike had the clips but I pinched the bicycle to travel to a variety of schools and supply teach. Not the most rewarding way of teaching but it kept my hand in and generated much needed income.

It was at this time that we decided to go and purchase a dog. This had always been a desire of ours—Mike particularly wanting a Golden Retriever because of childhood associations. We had admired a fine specimen of a dog whilst walking around Milton Keynes and stopping the owner, we discovered the name and details of a breeder. Mike promptly phoned to discover that she was, after a fashion, expecting a litter! We earmarked a puppy for ourselves. Excitement!

We travelled cross country to view this little puppy at five weeks; purchased and brought the little bundle of fur home at eight. Assured of her long-term temperament by the breeder, we planned to have her trained and organized ready for the arrival of our first child. Then baby and dog could grow up together, providing inseparable companionship for one another. Such stuff are dreams made of.

The puppy was named 'Dileas' (pronounced geelass). The name itself? Scottish Gaelic for 'faithful' in recognition of my Scottish connections. Suggested by my mother, Mike thought discretion the better part of valour and instantly agreed! In truth, we both fell in love with the name instantly and were most grateful to Mummy for introducing us to it. We did draw some old fashioned looks, however, when calling the dog to heel whilst walking in public parks! In time the name was vulgarized to 'Weely Woo' for some strange and unaccountable reason.

I expected to be at home to look after the puppy but no sooner had we purchased her than I was offered and accepted a term's full-time supply at a local middle school—covering for maternity leave! My turn next!

DIARY

May 1980 Mike kept me awake most of the night with a most ferocious hacking cough. He's plugging on regardless in his normal battling way but I for one am worried. When he gets a coughing fit, he gasps for air and is totally incapacitated.

June 1980 The cough continues. Energy is diminished—if not totally departed. Appetite for work also appears to have waned considerably—he must be struggling! I feel helpless; what should I do? Prayer of little apparent effect. Still summer's on the way, with a retreat and maybe some woman or man of God will have some insight.

Mind occupied with declining husband. Babies will have to wait—Mike has no energy for sex. Strange but I don't mind—I'm totally absorbed in his condition. I feel helpless; wish I could help. Powerless.

He's increasingly short tempered. Mustn't take what he says personally. Am finding the pressure intense. Great big 'HELP ME, GOD' prayers. Why don't the doctors have the important answers? Would we get better service with private health care? Totally in the hands of the medical profession. Mike really is low.

June 1980 Official verdict—off work. Mike has no energy for anything! The dog is the saving grace. He can spend all his time and what energy he has training her. This keeps him from insanity, I trust. Come to think of it, he's always been insane!

June 1980 Further tests. Mike returned to announce with great pride that he had Olympic lungs! How many more hospital visits? When will they have a fuller answer than the wretched word 'virus'? Still, at least we have plenty of time together for walking, talking, simply enjoying each other. I really enjoy chatting things over with Mike. He's even convincing me I've a brain and have original thoughts!

July 1980 Further prayer. Mike certainly acknowledged feelings of having been hurt on a number of occasions; also a fair amount of resentment and criticism is surfacing, mostly from

past experiences. Makes a clean break with them
by means of confession. Spiritual realm so hard to
relate to because the action comes from the un-
seen Spirit of God. We are so used to being in
charge of our own destiny. Trust this will all prove
helpful. Mike certainly seems brighter. Obser-
vation: physical problems may well have spiritual
roots—I must try to remember this.

COMMENTARY

Mike was not fit enough for work for six months.
He believed he should leave BYFC but made a
somewhat loaded deal with God. It was the
summer of the Ashes—England playing cricket
against Australia for the uninitiated. The third
test was at Headingly in Leeds. England looked all
but defeated at the close of the fourth day's play.
Indeed, to have survived that far was a surprise
both to the England team and the watching world.
The odds for an England victory at that stage
were 500-1 against!

Mike off work, and therefore forced to watch
cricket all day, arose Tuesday morning and
prayed:

'Father, if England win I'll stay in BYFC Amen.'

Mike felt sure that he was on his way to the
pavilion to begin looking for a new job. Yet as he
sat in front of the TV screen, a miracle occurred
before his very eyes. For only the second time in
test history, the side following on won the match.

England were delirious with delight. The pundits all amazed. The newspapers barely knew how to report it. Yet Mike, knowing differently, turned again to prayer and quietly agreed with God to continue his work with BYFC.

Neither of us advocate 'fleece laying' as a sure and certain method of guidance and yet must bear testimony to one of the most remarkable 'fleece' stories we know. Perhaps it speaks more of a truly remarkable God. A God who is truly supernatural and the boss. I leave it to the theologians to discuss the implications for Australia!

In spite of such exciting therapy, Mike's energy level did not noticeably improve. It is very difficult to maintain patience with someone who does not appear to be that ill outwardly. When walking to and from the paper shop, then reading the news, is sufficient to drain an individual of all their strength, it is very hard to relate to them. I contained my frustration and my emotions swung from overwhelming love and compassion to feeling totally disconcerted and wanting to scream at Mike to recover his former 'get up and go'. The issue was much more my felt insecurity within the situation than any animosity towards Mike. I relied upon him and now I was having to take all the decisions and I didn't like it. I am not an initiator and yet now I was cast in that role and needed to take it seriously. As week gave way to week, month to month, there were moments when I silently cried out from within, knowing I couldn't off-load all I was feeling on Mike and yet not knowing where else to turn.

However, were anyone to criticize Mike, I was the first to spring to his defence. I knew he felt somewhat of an abject failure. All his life he had achieved and now he lacked the strength to do whatever tasks he set for himself. Emotionally and spiritually this was draining him. I could almost see the fire dying in his eyes and his personal sense of failure writ large across his face. Often so called helpful advice from those classing themselves as friends drove him into deeper distress. Like the suggestion that he simply pull himself together! offered at the end of a time of counsel set up not by Mike but the person who concluded their in-depth considerations with that statement.

DIARY

August 1980 EYEMOUTH. Six miles north of Berwick on the east coast of Scotland. A place filled with childhood memories from numerous happy holidays. Mike's first visit; hope he likes it. Condition stabilized. I'd hardly believe Mike needed a holiday but he is lacking in energy still. A good rest, and a good read; the usual way for recharging his batteries. However, what if the batteries are not rechargeable?

August 1980 Mike loves the place—I'm thrilled. Endless card and board games; ambling around the active harbour; nothing in particular but Mike is coping with it all very well.

Making love again; it's good. Mike's impotency appears to have passed. Why no one ever told us before we married that stress could induce periods of impotency I just can't think. I've never seen anyone so dejected as Mike when he was simply unable to make love. Certainly learnt that a man's self-esteem, ego, etc is very directly related to his sexual ability. Mike also feared that my love, respect and commitment for him would diminish. No amount of affirmation appeared to penetrate his thick skull. Obstinate bloke at times. Still, the Scottish air must have done the trick; rampant insecurity gives way to rampant sexuality!

August 1980 St Francis of Assisi used to give everything in life the name of an animal it resembled—the human body he termed 'Brother Ass'. I believe the act of sex must be a prime example of this most fitting description. It is good to be making love again—strange expression 'to make love'—and with Mike almost chirpy once again, I am sure I shall be pregnant soon. Certainly, my mind is once again focused upon children and I really long for them. I am waiting with eager anticipation and with a fair measure of expectation for the end of the month and no period. That in itself would be a blessing especially to avoid the pain barrier I must go through each time. Seems to me men got the best bargain out of the fall! There again, God knew best. The human race would have ceased long ago if men had been the child bearers; I am amazed at the negligible pain threshold of most men.

CHAPTER ONE

COMMENTARY

The end of the month came and went. I was not pregnant. Those same period pains were by November so strong that I went to visit the doctor for his advice. It made a change for the doctor to see me and not Mike. Mike's condition was much improved, though his return to work was delayed by an ingrowing toe nail which required removal with root to prevent repetition.

It was also one year since we had started trying to conceive and I took the opportunity to air the subject with the doctor. He listened intently and sympathetically before pointing out that, with all that Mike had been through, it was hardly conducive to becoming pregnant. We were to learn a lot about the lack of pressure and the incidence of pregnancy through our talks with various medics.

While I accepted all this at face value, I felt deeply disappointed inside. I suppose I really wanted an immediate answer or at the very least, to be assured that all was well and that—hey presto—I would be pregnant next month. There were more nagging doubts about the likelihood of my becoming pregnant than I had realized through the period of looking after Mike.

The doctor, a Christian, obviously read between the lines. In response to my anxiety, he suggested Mike should undergo a couple of sperm counts to ensure that he wasn't firing blanks! I left the surgery armed with hospital forms, plastic bottles and a sense of relief as well as devastation. Relief in that we had something to do and didn't just have to mark time month by month, hoping that my period would fail to materialize. Devastation in that a step had been taken and the door marked 'Infertility' pushed open just a fraction. I was afraid of what I might discover if once I stepped through that door. I could not bear the thought that Mike and I would not be able to have children.

Chapter Two

DIARY

January 1981 Strange how one can't avoid the issue God is dealing with—or wanting to deal with. Got to know a couple through church contact: John and Maria. They live some distance away but we get on well and Maria seems to have limpet-like qualities—she sticks to me like glue. Being a friendly, hospitable and at home lady of leisure, I gladly extend the hand of friendship.

January 1981 The ladies' meeting. That time of the week when some unassuming individual carelessly opens her home to receive the women from the church, many with offspring in tow. Amidst the learned exposition of Scripture by one of the number—or on special occasions, a guest—the children gladly co-operate by playing together, successfully tipping orange juice on the settee, crushing well-gummed biscuits into the carpet, breaking the heads off the beautifully arranged vaseful of flowers. Running out of such entertaining pursuits, they turn their attention to brutalizing each other, and delightful gurgles of glee are replaced by screams of tortured infants. This signals the group leader to turn hastily to prayer and bring the meeting to a close. How did Jesus teach the crowds when the local kids declared war on each other? This would prove an interesting study.

I take Maria with me. During the procedures, I notice her getting increasingly uptight. Is there heresy being preached? I think not: the arrangements for the next church social may appear horrifying but they're unlikely to lead to ex-communication.

Coffee arrives—took the opportunity to ask Maria if she was OK. Bad move; hit raw nerve; emotions flow from her eyes and roll down her cheeks. I invite her for lunch to get the full story. Lunch agreed for the following day. I've a feeling Maria and I have some miles to travel together. Feel a measure of inadequacy, interest, expectation and frustration. Now is not the time to psychoanalyse my reaction to hearing and responding to other people's woes. As Mike would say, 'Go to it, kid!' I shall.

January 1981 Maria for lunch (after a manner of speaking, you understand!) The full story is told. After five years of marriage, John and Maria

decide to start a family. Both have proved successful at work—they have a fine home base and
the financial security to provide for a family.
Conceiving fairly quickly all looked good until
Maria miscarried, an experience which she found
traumatic and hard to recover from. Advised to
wait for three months before trying to conceive
again, they were now two years down the road
from the miscarriage and Maria was still not
pregnant. Didn't tell her of our situation since we
were keeping fairly *stumm* about it.

My only response to this harrowing history was
to mouth simple platitudes such as 'it's only a
matter of time' and 'you'll be all right'—about as
handy as a hammer to a precision watchmaker!

August 1981 We lunched with John and Maria. A
good time: learnt an excellent new card game to
add to our repertoire; it will need re-titling, however.

Good to get to know John and Maria as a
couple. John is an exceptionally caring husband.
Thanked me for being Maria's friend. I only hope
I deserve the thanks; I'm not sure how effective a
friend I'm proving.

From our conversations, it is evident that childlessness dominates Maria's life—her every waking
thought is children. When she meets children, she
always reacts: cries, leaves their vicinity or retreats
into herself. No wonder she's quiet at the ladies
meeting.

Evening Mike and I talk about our time with

John and Maria. We want to be friends to them but feel totally at a loss to know how to respond. Suppose we must just play it by ear. I shall make myself available to Maria as and when she needs me. We agreed to pray for them and the desire of their hearts, namely, children. I also felt anxious that if I remained childless, would my life follow the same pattern as Maria's? Day closed with prayer.

COMMENTARY

Little did I realize what it would mean making myself available to Maria. I soon learned that, having always been personally successful at all she had undertaken, not to become pregnant, which appeared one of the most natural processes in life, was well nigh impossible for her to accept. She felt a failure and so had to learn to cope with the emotions, etc sparked off by that sense of failure. Not being in control was a very real pressure and problem to her. Whenever we were together, which was very often, the issue of childlessness dominated the conversation. No matter what diversionary tactics I introduced—shopping trips, sightseeing, topics of current interest—infertility remained the dominant theme. I had never in my life seen anyone so absorbed with one issue.

Very quickly, I realized that I was needed very much as a sounding board—someone to be talked at rather than expected to give verbal response. If

I did offer an opinion, Maria was not capable of weighing it up; it almost appeared to pass her by, like water running off a duck's back.

I discovered she was seeing a variety of people with the explicit purpose of receiving 'counsel'. Some of these were Christian counsellors, some secular. This ensured she was subject to conflicting advice, yet being desperate for an escape from her nightmare, she attempted to respond to it all. The result was chaos and confusion. Should I attempt to give advice? I felt sure it would only confuse her totally, so limited myself to attempts at enabling her to make sense of all the counsel she was receiving. This was no easy matter as advice flowed from glib Christian triumphalism— i.e. Jesus is the answer, pull yourself together, live in victory, etc—to Freudian therapy—i.e. God is a big 'ought' which dominates Maria's life and the first step to relaxing in order to conceive is to ditch God and stop trying to live relating to him.

However, I do believe my role of practical support was vital, a role I was regularly encouraged in by John. Evidently, because Maria was so hypersensitive as well as consumed with childlessness, it had not been easy for her to sustain friendships, to the extent that when you put together those people from whose company Maria excluded herself because of the close proximity of children with those who found her sole topic of conversation and emotional state too overbearing, you had more or less listed all of the church. While from the outside looking in, it is easy to see why people who are so totally locked into a personal issue are difficult to build a friendship with and easier avoided, experiencing childlessness myself I have discovered how isolating an experience it can be. Somehow bridgeheads need to be established so that the childless couple are never totally lost sight of, for there is a common path down which they all must walk. Like Jesus on the Emmaus Road, they all need someone, a stranger perhaps, to fall in step alongside them, to be their friend and re-focus their eyes on Jesus at regular intervals.

I was also to learn how readily Christians will offer their thoughts on the matter, often in the guise of counsel, take offence if it is not received appropriately, yet totally forget they ever said anything by failing to enquire if there is any real fruit from their words so easily spoken. I very quickly learnt with Maria that my role was support and that I could keep superfluous advice to myself. It would be true to say that I am grateful to Maria to this day for teaching me so much about being a friend to a hurting person—I trust she holds similarly warm regards for my bumbling attempt in that direction.

As time went on, Maria did become a pressure as far as I was concerned. She would arrive unannounced at the house; sometimes spend all day with me, not wanting to be on her own, and only returning home once John was back from work. It was through this process, I learned a lot about handling people; setting specific time limits for our meeting together; initiating activities; learning to be direct, yet kind, in saying what I felt without fearing the immediate reaction that could follow. However, I also found this totally draining and did not have the encouragement of any noticeable changes in Maria.

When eventually I confessed that Mike and I were having problems conceiving, it was incredible how I heard my own insipid platitudes spoken back to me. They were of no more encouragement to me than they had obviously been to Maria. I did find it difficult not to slip into self-pity myself on occasions, every fibre in my being wanting to shout out, 'But what about me? I can't have children either! It's not just your problem!' Indeed, after a while, it began to magnify my own anxieties with regard to childlessness—all of which I found very depressing.

We continued to see Maria and John until we left the area. Not long afterwards, we received a letter telling us of her pregnancy and a little later another announcing the arrival of a baby. I was both thrilled for them and desperately disappointed for us. It seemed ironic that our prayers for them had apparently been heard and acted upon, while those for ourselves were bouncing back unheeded as if to mock us. And yet one only had to turn in the Bible to Genesis and discover Abraham praying for the harem of Abimelech who—owing to an unfortunate oversight on Abraham's part in failing to introduce Sarah as his wife for fear of being murdered by some who were lustful and infatuated with her beauty—were made infertile by God (Gen 20: 1–18). His prayer was successful in removing this short-term barrenness and yet he and Sarah continued in their own childlessness for a number of years. In fact, when God finally told Abraham his wife would conceive, the conversation was interrupted by giggles emanating from the tent where Sarah sat listening in, as she found it both impossible and hilarious to believe a woman of her advanced years should conceive—and yet she did and I suppose she was privileged to over-hear the hilarity in heaven as she announced her pregnancy to Abraham!

Although I had returned from the doctor's the previous November ready to press forward with infertility tests, the forms and bottles for Mike's sperm counts lay idle for five months. Concerned that investigations were beginning, I was more upset that things had to begin with Mike. Irrationally, I wanted the difficulty to be on my side—to this day I don't know why. I also half believed that the moment we initiated tests, I would immediately become pregnant—a sort of superstition that abounds. Indeed, many folk encouraged us in that way once they knew of our situation or the other old chestnut: 'Once you adopt a child, you'll have one of your own!' It appears to us that 90% of the people we meet know someone who became pregnant just after adopting a child. Of course, the underlying principle is superstition—we'll adopt a baby in order to conceive ourselves—hardly a godly attitude. It's an attitude which also keeps one from facing the issue square on. There is a great lack of realism surrounding subjects such as childlessness, and failing to look the problem full in the face helps neither partner nor couple. One constantly wants to live in hope, which is no bad thing unless that hope is any straw eagerly grasped as the waters of despair rise in a vain attempt to avoid drowning. Swimming has to do with giving oneself to the water, not thrashing around unsuccessfully to be free of it. Equally, childlessness can only begin to be coped with as both partners individually and together acknowledge openly their situation, express honestly the emotions in the light of this and together determine how they will not simply stay afloat but actually engage in a purposeful stroke. This will entail taking hold of their experience of infertility and weaving it effectively into the tapestry of their life together. All this is clear to us now but as we engaged in the first steps towards infertility testing, we were also entering a hard school of learning— grateful that we knew that right along with us was God himself, an ever-present help in times of trouble.

DIARY

March 1982 Period started today. Feel very depressed and very angry. Why is it all the pregnant teenagers we talk with courtesy of Youth for Christ have only a one night stand to blame for it? We've been unsuccessful with eighteen months of one night stands! Period pain intense but fortunately the 'yellow torpedoes', prescribed by the doctor, certainly do the trick. I must broach the subject of childlessness with Mike again.

March 1982 Evening together. Short of finance, so low-budget evening meal. Candle in milk bottle captures the Bohemian poverty in a most expensive way. Lifts the status of shepherd's pie to something on a par with salmon mousse! We dress for dinner to give it a sense of occasion. Unfortunately, the wine waiter—a handsome lad looking very much like my husband—spilt grape juice (the wine cellar being unfortunately empty) down Mike's fine white shirt. Really proving difficult to get the right quality of service these days.

The meal over, coffee in hand, we lounge luxuriously on the settee and chat. I bring the conversation around to babies—Mike is all too ready to talk it through. A wave of relief runs through me. It's so difficult to know when Mike is feeling raw and the subject itself then causes him to tense up. But this evening we can talk and plan. We agree the sperm count must be done over the next week.

March 1982 Sperm count number one. I never realized how great a mental barrier there was for Mike in this. All he had to do was produce sperm for analysis—or so I thought. However, I watched him go through a fair degree of emotional anxiety. Partly fear that the test would prove that he was unable to father children. Partly embarrassment at having to do the test at all.

Once he had produced a specimen, he asked me to take it up to the clinic—too embarrassed to hand it in to the female receptionist. He's always honest. There is a measure of farce to all this, since the specimen dies after a certain amount of time, so all must be co-ordinated with the arrival of the hospital van at the doctor's surgery. We laughed at this—if a little nervously—to help handle the whole situation. I see that Mike really does find the whole problem very painful. Also it means coming to terms with one's sexuality.

Delivered sperm sample safely, and in time, at the doctor's. In the guise of a courier I leapt on to my push-bike and pedalled furiously to the clinic. Bottled and tastefully sealed in an NHS brown envelope, the specimen bounced along very happily in the basket on the front of the bicycle. Handing it over, the thought passed through my mind 'one sperm specimen, shaken not stirred!'

Talked to Mike about the situation this evening. He said he found it hard to masturbate mechanically in the interests of medicine. He found it all too clinical and scientific. Mike hates a de-personalized world, as he states on numerous occasions.

Masturbation—an interesting subject for Christians. Q. When is masturbation not masturbation? A. When it's in the interests of a sperm count?

COMMENTARY

That was the first of two sperm counts. Before the second, Mike had to wait three days and then one week for the results. There was plenty of activity since we were getting ready for Spring Harvest where Mike and I were leading TOSH, the programme for the fifteen- to eighteen-year-olds on site. This entailed taking responsibility for a team of youth workers, as well as the programme content and its smooth running.

When the time for the second sperm count came, Mike dutifully went to the bathroom, bottle in hand. I waited to speed this second specimen up the road to the clinic. Nothing ever runs to plan. At that moment the doorbell rang and our friend Christine Rumbol, the minister's daughter, was on the doorstep. I showed her into the lounge; Mike appeared, slipped the brown paper envelope with its live cargo into my hand and I made an excuse and pedalled off, leaving Mike to chat to Christine. When I returned home, the coffee was made and I joined in the conversation feeling very furtive. I'm sure I could never make a secret agent, I'd never stay the pace or cope with the intrigue.

We were keen to get the results and the waiting seemed unendurably long. Mike was glad to have got the tests out of the way. I found myself hoping with all my might that they would prove good. The last thing I wanted, as I've said before, was for Mike to be infertile. It has proved interesting to meet infertile couples since that time and dis-

cover how often the husbands will not initiate tests
of themselves. It seems as though the struggles
Mike had within himself are far from unique.
And yet a sperm count is so simple and easy a
test—and to be honest, statistics demonstrate that
90% of males masturbate and the other 10% are
lying!—that not to take it is a very selfish attitude.
Should it prove that the individual has a low
sperm count, then as a couple as well as with
others, conversations need to take place to assure
the man that his sexuality and his essential
'himness' is in no way diminished. There is so very
little teaching in the church today on positive
sexuality, something so necessary in the face of
the vast market in sex and sexual roles in society
today. Television fantasy portrayed as reality
is dictating role models to generation after
generation; role models that are non-biblical yet
go unchallenged by the church, save for out-
breaks of moral outrage. Yet the church has very
clear models revealed through Scripture. Young
people are desperate to hear these described and,
through the marriages they observe, to see such
demonstrated. Unless this happens, they will consistently choose sexual promiscuity as the only
valid expression of sexuality for that is apparently
all that is on offer; all that they can observe. My
plea to all husbands of infertile couples would be
that they take the necessary tests—it is wanton
cruelty not to for two reasons. In the first place, if
it means infertility is never explored from a medical angle, one of the keenest desires in a woman
must be suppressed in this case by your wife.

Proverbs 30: 15–16 states:

> There are three things that are never satisfied,
> Four that never say, 'Enough!':
> The grave, the barren womb,
> Land, which is never satisfied with water,
> And fire, which never says, 'Enough!'

Scripture is clear that barrenness is something one has to learn to live with but which will always, I believe, carry a deep-felt ache which cannot be satisfied. Not to take what steps are available in identifying the problem is to add the unnecessary pain and pressure of not knowing if the situation is simply rectified or not. Many infertile couples are swiftly and effectively treated by the NHS.

Secondly, there is no pain whatsoever in a sperm count—(rather, pleasure at the physical level!). There is emotional anxiety. However, the woman will usually need a laparoscopy for starters, at the very least entailing an overnight hospital stay, general anaesthetic and a degree of physical discomfort. If any husband is prepared unnecessarily to put his wife through such a process, I personally would like to bop him on the nose, and what's more, I know Mike would join me.

We got the results of Mike's tests the day before we departed for Spring Harvest. They proved a mixed blessing. One was fine the other was, quote: 'a little dubious'. This meant a re-run. Mike groaned inwardly—I did outwardly. Yet we were determined to put the whole subject out of our minds for the duration of Spring Harvest and throw ourselves into the work whole-heartedly.

On our return, the tests were repeated—further embarrassment for Mike; more secret-agent activities for me! We were both relieved when the results came back and all was well. Certainly Mike could father children. But now the spotlight swung across the stage and fixed its beady eye on me. Would I be able to conceive and carry children?

I needed some time for quiet reflection and took the dog for a walk. My emotions were in a whirl. They fired so many contradictory messages to my brain that I found myself in a state of confusion: I was thrilled that Mike was clear, but what of me? There's more chance of a medical solution this way round I calmly told myself. But what would tests mean? An internal was bad enough! I knew Mike would be supportive. But what if I couldn't give him the children he now knew he could father?

It was as if I was watching a piece of cinema action with the pressure on me to retain all the details I observed, ready to face the rapid-fire questioning of some imaginary game-show host. The adrenalin was pumping, I was keyed up and as each new thought thrust its way into my mind, I found myself desperately seeking to retain a grip on the previous one. All my powers of self-control came into play in order that I might not become the object of my mind's activity. Rather, I fought to return to being the subject of my own life by quoting aloud—'O! that way madness lies; let me shun that'—after the fashion of Shakespeare's

47

King Lear. However, one verbal aversion does not necessarily shape the course of one's life, as I was to discover. The power of positive thinking can lead to bankruptcy.

On returning home, I discovered Mike had also been doing some GBH (grievous brain harm) and the fruit of it was expressed by, firstly, sitting me down, secondly, supplying me with a cup of tea and some chocolate (how precious chocolate is at moments of crisis!) and finally lifting the weight of responsibility from my shoulders by saying: 'Let's go at the pace we can cope with and no faster. You call the shots and I'll action the decisions. Deal?'

'Deal!' I said, gratefully melting into his arms, covering the sleeves of his arran jumper with soft chocolate and salty tears. As usual, he took it in good part with no more than a patient sigh!

Chapter Three

Milton Keynes—new city—a shopping precinct
provides a cathedral to encourage worship of the
modern-day god of materialism, is to my mind
instantly forgettable. New housing estate gives
way to newer housing estate with monotonous
regularity and recently planted saplings indicate a
tree-lined future, probably at a point in time
when even the newest housing estate will have
given way to weeds, nettles and the encroachment
of nature. Once one has experienced the excitement of concrete cows and the reality of Great
Linford (the one scenic part of Milton Keynes,
fully exploited by the advertisers on hoardings
enticing beleaguered London city dwellers to the
nirvana of country living with all labour-saving
amenities), there is not much left to inspire. Built
for the two-car family, the carless are poorly
catered for since the chaotic bus service struggles

to provide any kind of reasonable service from the outlying estate to the city centre.

As for the weather, there is a tiring, relentless wind which blows throughout the year. When Mike and I first moved to Milton Keynes in November 1980, we awoke the following morning to find snow on the ground! Yes, in November! Keen to discover our new surroundings, we determined to walk to the city centre—a journey of around forty-five minutes we were assured. Wrapping up warmly, we set out along the cycle paths (without the cycles), which prevented one from coming into contact with motorized transport on the roads. The temperature appeared to be polar and the wind cut like a knife. Bent double, we pressed on, walking into the teeth of the gale. The further we went, the colder we got and the more beleagured we felt. My mind recalled Captain Scott's trip in Antarctica—and I was not at all convinced we would make it. Eventually, we sighted civilization on the horizon. A complex structure of metal and glass rising stark-like from the concrete surrounds of roads, bridges, pedestrian areas and flats. Dragging ourselves across a large, enclosed piazza, we finally collapsed in the restaurant of John Lewis, gratefully drank hot—oh, delightfully hot—coffee and slowly thawed out, too exhausted to talk. The journey home was equally gruelling—our welcome to Milton Keynes, city of dreaming town planners (I wish someone had woken them before the plans left the drawing board).

Milton Keynes, city of Mike's illness, where the

doctor's surgery became familiar to us both and where I began to look for an answer to my infertility, joining what has become the modern day preoccupation with medical answers for inconvenient physical problems.

One of the delights of wanting to start a family is that one can forget all about contraception. I had enjoyed an early introduction to the contraceptive Pill. As a teenager, I had suffered acute period pains. I well remember giving a speech at school as deputy head girl, well laced with vodka to control the excruciating pain I was enduring, it being the inconvenient time of the month. The doctor assured me in prescribing the Pill that such treatment would suppress ovulation and therefore eliminate all pain. Glory, alleluia, I thought (or would have done had I been a convinced Christian); in the event, I settled for yabadabadoo! If only investigation had been made at that stage, perhaps my condition would have been diagnosed earlier. And yet, 'Regrets are idle, yet history is one long regret. Everything might have turned out so differently' (Charles Duddley Warner). Certainly, I enjoyed the benefit of no period pain—and the advantage of 'safe' sex should I desire it in my teenage years (safe in the sense of avoiding pregnancy!).

When Mike and I got married, we opted for the Pill as the easiest form of contraception. Mike had suggested a glass of water—not before, not after, but instead of! However, in the event our passions were not to be thwarted and the Pill it was. Once we decided we wanted a family, the doctor advised that we take steps to prevent conception for the first three months after stopping the Pill to allow all the residue to clear from my body. It was at this point that we opted for the sheath—a form of contraception that we tried on a couple of occasions but detested so much that the three months were spent in abstention rather than endure what Mike has termed 'one of the most unpleasant experiences of my life.' It was the overwhelming smell of rubber and what Mike perceived as lack of intimacy—depersonalization after a fashion. I recount our experience only to demonstrate that contraception is a very personal thing—well, sex is really come to that—and it is for us as couples to work out our own preferences.

Having attempted sex 'crowd stopper' fashion, we began to discuss the future. What would we do after we had our family, or more especially, what would we do to space out our children and avoid producing one a year? Mike was quite happy to have a vasectomy once the family was complete—this is, of course, the easiest and simplest solution and removes the anguish of possible pregnancy. We have met a number of couples who have the children they want, whose budgets are stretched to cope with a growing family and who fear that their chosen form of contraception may fail, leaving them to face a further pregnancy and another child. This situation has produced stress for the couple, a stress that has communicated itself to the existing children, producing tension and insecurity within the family home. The reason given most frequently is that should one or other of the partners die and the surviving member choose to remarry, they would not want to be in the position of being unable to produce children with their new partner. We see this as the most convoluted thinking, only surpassed by the cry of the male ego claiming that a vasectomy in some way reduces his manhood. My only comment would be, did he have any manhood in the first place? If vasectomy removes manhood, when the act of intercourse can still be undertaken without fear of inadvertent pregnancy, then what is this manhood that ends its life under the surgeon's knife?

Vasectomy is such a simple operation and, even if a trifle humiliating, embarrassing and painful, can hardly compare with the ordeal women are expected to endure in playing their part in the procreation process. Fathers take note, ask not to whom the surgeon's knife beckons, it beckons to you!

However, we had no family as yet but, fully expecting to produce, the key decision was what form of contraception to use to space out the children? It was at this stage that I talked long and hard to an old school friend of mine. Joanna had married Nigel, a good friend of Mike's, a week after our own wedding. In fact, we had returned from our honeymoon in exotic Exeter to participate in their nuptial celebrations. Joanna and Nigel were both Catholics and took the church's teaching on contraception seriously. As a result, they were to practise natural family planning. I had heard of the rhythm method, often derisively described as 'Russian roulette', but was amused to discover how scientific it actually was. Joanna lent me a number of books on the subject and I went and purchased an ovulation thermometer from the chemist. Mike and I decided to practise natural family planning while we were wanting to conceive. If I became pregnant, we would be delighted, while monitoring my temperature would also give us an indication of the most propitious time for love-making each month.

Joanna also directed me to write to the Catholic Family Planning Association (CFPA). This agency had trained counsellors around the country who helped couples with the finer points of natural family planning or Billings Method as it was also called, after Dr Billings, a gynaecologist who had pioneered a great deal in this area. Before I could write, a series of coincidences intervened.

In Milton Keynes we attended the local ecumenical centre—Anglican, Methodist and Baptist worshipping together, preceeded by the Catholics. I suppose this is ecumenism in action. It was not a style of worship or church life that either Mike or I particularly enjoyed but there were some interesting people involved. Although the Catholics and Protestants met separately throughout the year, we did all come together to study during Lent. It was during this Lenten course that I met Veronica, a nun from a local convent; we were in the same small group together and got on particularly well. I've always believed myself to be an exceptionally hospitable person but over coffee at the end of the evening, no sooner had I introduced Mike than Sister Veronica invited us both to the convent for an evening meal and to meet the other nuns—an invitation we readily accepted.

Arriving at the convent, a name describing the function of a large house in the north of the city, we were greeted by Sister Veronica before being introduced to the 'boss'—the Mother Superior, Sister Angela. She was a delightful woman with a radiant smile and eyes that flashed as though flames flickered in their depths. We received a most infectious welcome and were immediately at ease with this lovely group of caring ladies. So relaxed were we that during the evening, I found myself explaining to Sister Angela our great desire for children and the difficulties we might face in this area. I also told of our interest in natural family planning. What possessed me to speak so openly about sex to an avowed celibate, I do not know. In any case my honesty was rewarded with the discovery that Sister Angela was one of the counsellors for the CFPA, which Joanna had told me about. Without further ado, I made arrangements to visit Sister Angela one afternoon and we left very happy with our evening.

The whole subject of natural family planning is fascinating. Mention it to the ordinary person off the street and they find it all highly amusing and quite unbelievable. I was, however, to meet couples who had ordered the size of their families by employing this method. Obviously, there were those unexpected surprises but I've also discovered that in the case of couples utilizing the contraceptive Pill! It was also fascinating to learn that a full course on this method was run at Birmingham University, a course which Sister Angela herself was enrolled in and which she all but convinced me to attend.

As I have mentioned, I was beginning to use an ovulation thermometer. Sister Angela explained that to comprehend fully the menstrual cycle, a woman must be aware of her temperature and mucus—hence natural family planning should more accurately be termed the thermo-muco method or thermo-nuclear as Mike dubbed it! I was given a great sheaf of charts and Mike, who was with me (and to give him his due, has taken a deep personal interest in all the activities related to infertility throughout), was given his instructions by a kind but firm Mother Superior. He would have to make the early morning cup of tea while I lay in bed and took my temperature. I was not allowed either to move or drink anything prior to this activity. Having read the thermometer, I was to plot the result on one of the charts, each of which covered a calendar month.

Alongside this activity, I had to learn to recognize and read the various mucus secretions from my vagina. These were termed 'cloudy', 'sticky' and 'egg-white' and once identified, I made a note of this on my monthly chart. Though some readers may find this difficult to believe or find it an exceptionally laborious process, I was unwittingly producing a bank of information which was to prove invaluable to the doctors who later treated my infertility. I was able to provide them with an eighteen-month record of my ovulation pattern—indeed, the charts themselves demonstrated I was ovulating, and regularly! Had I not had the material to hand, I would have had to take a number of months generating such information. Besides all that, it gave me something new to focus my mind on. Anything new provided a source of hope and encouragement. If this was not the answer *per se*, it certainly set Mike and me on the path to successful conception, or so I liked to muse. Fortunately, we are both suckers for gimmicks and 'newness' and so Mike joined in this new dimension to love-making with enthusiasm, even accompanying me to the library to order the books on the Billings Method. He never actually read them, however, preferring historical-biography throughout!

DIARY

March 1982 A new day dawns; a new move beckons. Go north, young man! Mike is to go to Leeds in his work for BYFC. He will act as co-ordinator for the North. The job description has obviously been designed by an Englishman, for his brief is the North of England AND Scotland! If you chop along the line of the border between the two kingdoms and superimpose Scotland on England, it comes down as far as London! Not a lot of people know that; none apparently in

BYFC. Mike will certainly have a big patch. Fortunately, we've been given a car by my brother —however, even the thought of all that mileage in a Fiat 126 with 60,000 on the clock already causes me some heart-stopping anxiety. Gird up thy loins and pack, dear girl, now is not the time for idle speculation.

May 1982 Refreshed reading the Bible today. Praying on and off about childless situation— funny how so pressing an issue fails to be the subject of my prayer life every day. Perhaps I am not that concerned really, although I feel most concerned. Maybe I'm faithless, a sort of also-ran Christian. I've a prayer but not quite the energy or passion to pursue it relentlessly. Reading Psalms—113: 9 to be precise—the following words made a particular impression upon me: 'He settles the barren woman in her home as the happy mother of children.' Took hold of that phrase and found great encouragement. Perhaps our move to Leeds will prove a little more permanent than our housing to date. This may provide my 'home'—would like somewhere to feel I belong and time to 'play houses' and turn it into more than just an abode.

Told Mike of my encouragement from the Bible—typical reply: 'Ah, birds of the air have nests and foxes holes . . .' Before he finished, I was wiping the wicked grin off his face with a well moistened dish cloth. Emerging from a scrum of flailing arms and legs, he took time to encourage me. The rat—but I love him. Why?

May 1982 Agree to work formally with Mike as his secretary. Accompany him on a preaching engagement and discover why he was so keen for me to take on the job. Tells congregation he enjoys sleeping with his secretary, who also happens to be his wife. When I'm an international celebrity, I'll studiously avoid introducing him to all the interesting people I meet, while insisting he keep in tow with me!

May 1982 Strange how people will not leave messages for Mike with me. Having explained I'm his secretary, they obviously believe me to be somewhat brainless and uninformed. Mike's travelling a lot now—finding the days very long. Wake in the mornings with only my thermometer to kiss. It consistently refuses to return my affection. Chart-keeping something of a chore now. Will wait till we move before taking investigations further. Thought of bringing another doctor up to date with 'the story so far' does not warm the cockles of my heart.

News of the safe arrival of Jane's baby—jars somewhat. Am pleased and jealous at the same time. I know that I can get a grip of such jealousy —the issue is, do I want to?

June 1982 The move. Removal men arrive early —a cheerful bunch. Disturbing to see one's familiar life packed away in boxes. Strike a deal with removers: cup of tea on the hour every hour in return for suitable photo-call on van. Good photo—good to embarrass Mike! All loaded swiftly. All the odd bits of timber, etc collected by Mike because 'they might come in useful some-day' prove a problem. Everything going into storage for a week, so have to sign inventory of everything loaded.

Wave van farewell. One last tour of house—pleased to be leaving a place with few happy memories but reticent about stepping away from what has become the familiar. Drive to Wolverhampton to spend our 'homeless' week with Phil and Julie. A good time in prospect.

June 1982 Arrive Leeds—welcome removal van. Some of the team are the same as those who packed everything up for us. Great welcome from the local fellowship—Ken McGreavy and Ian Rowbottom come by to help unload. Confused by the amount of household furniture Mike consigns to the garage. Confirmed in their view that southerners are strange.

Once unloaded, ate the best tasting fish and chips ever and fell asleep on the sofa—so far so good!

June 1982 Locate doctor and register. Now the moment of truth; the time to take the infertility issue a stage further—the door opens wider; a long uninviting corridor stretches before me. Mike is alongside me but there will be places he will not be able to accompany me. I both steel myself for this journey and cry out to God for strength, help, encouragement and friendship. Will I make it? I certainly feel the pressure building. 'God go with me please—I've never felt so small, so over-whelmed, so inconsequential—my moorings have been cut and I'm adrift in a strange world I never wanted to visit. God go with me please. Amen.'

There can be few more depressing places to sit than a doctor's waiting room. Seated around the wall with a host of strangers, apart from those with sneezes and wheezes, one can only imagine what tales of ill health each has to recount. All hoping the doctor—often exalted to godhead in our modern world, with his apparent ability to heal, fulfilling the traditional role of witch-doctor of old—will provide a remedy. For some, he will pronounce a sentence of death.

Only the rustle of cast off magazines to disturb one's thoughts, poised to leap up at the appro-priate summons, I let my eye wander around these inauspicious surroundings. The walls, emulsioned pink some long time ago, showed the tell-tale signs of age; cracks running up the wall—paint flaking—colour insipid, as though the original brightness had all been sucked out. The chairs, an assortment of oddments, no doubt generously donated; all worn; most fairly upright and uncomfortable. The table on which the magazines were scattered bore the scars of hot drinks stood carelessly upon its polished wooden surface, and superficial gashes in the veneer. The carpet, threadbare and exhausted, appeared to have expired some years previously. The sixty-watt bulb in the light fitting suspended from the centre of the ceiling cast an unnatural light across the room, the heavy cotton curtains obscuring the day and helping to create the impression that one has stepped out of the world of work, leisure, laughter and friendship into another place altogether. Mike and I sat next to each other—me gazing around the room, Mike looking down at his feet, which he shuffled from time to time in an attempt both to pass the time and change the focus of his studied concentration.

We had been in this situation before. The expectation was for further medical tests—probably hospitalization for me. I knew Mike felt the pain of our situation keenly. However, a born activist, I realized the total sense of having no control over the situation aggravated him more. Here was my shining knight who had, by various means, always come to my aid and rescued me from the jaws of several dragons which were apparently due to devour me, who now found his weapons blunted and his courage frustrated by the nature of the challenge. This was to call for different traits. I wondered if Mike would actually find it within himself to get through.

For my part, I was glad we were at the doctor's. Mike had delayed and dragged his feet, not really wanting to come face to face with the expected medical conclusions. Somehow, he could cope with living in a state of perpetual suspended animation. I could not. I wanted to press ahead and surely the next visit, the ensuing test, would prove to be the final step in our quest to produce a family.

The buzzer brought me back to reality and I prodded Mike. We rose, crossed the floor and entered the surgery. We were greeted by a genial smile and word of welcome. The doctor, for this was my first visit to this particular practice, was obviously approaching retirement. He had a shock of white hair, a kindly face, well worn and wrinkled. My immediate impression was of a trusted grandpa figure. I felt reassured to be entrusting my deepest hopes and desires to him. Instinctively, I knew Mike was relaxing and had obviously taken to the doctor as well.

I knew I had to speak and shot an arrow prayer skyward and Godward in the hope that emotion would not rob me of my ability to communicate our situation. Fortunately, the doctor had cast his eye over our notes and hardly had I begun the explanation for our visit than he interrupted and gave us some advice which has stayed with us both ever since and proved fundamental in our experience together.

Sensing my rawness and vulnerability, the doctor provided what must be described as a pastoral chat. Acknowledging the pain we both must feel, he was at pains to point out that childlessness was a joint problem—a problem of the couple as a couple. He made it clear that it was neither one partner's nor the other's fault, although the physical disability might be traced to one party. If we were to handle realistically our apparent childlessness and successfully weather the further tests and investigations, we would need to agree together that this was our problem and neither attribute blame nor adopt a mantle of guilt. To do so, would be to do damage to our marriage.

These words were so wise. I do not believe we had in fact ever blamed each other or felt the pressure of undue guilt. However, this opinion provided a point from which we could ourselves talk the subject through with greater honesty. Indeed, the doctor in his wisdom began such a process by drawing a verbal response from us both to what he had outlined and gently engaged us in conversation with each other. I remain eternally grateful to a doctor who saw that behind a medical presenting problem, lay two whole human beings with minds and emotions and that the essential issue lay not in the presenting problem but in the very nature of our individual ability to cope with ourselves and each other. It was to prove a rarity to meet with medics who had the same capacity to see beyond and therefore treat more than the presenting problem!

COMMENTARY

The fruit of our visit was that a letter to the LGI (Leeds General Infirmary) would be written and sent. More than that, however, Mike and I had a clear task to talk through our childlessness honestly—not avoiding the issue for what it was. For me, I had to express my own insecurity about the fact that I was apparently unable to supply him with children of his own. Mike may choose to reject me. This could be emotionally by locking me out of his life, or physically by leaving and choosing another. One of the most heart-rending stories I had heard was where a childless couple, when the physical problem lay with the woman, had brought about a total breakdown in the marriage. The husband, unable to cope with the thought of not fathering his own children, had taken up with another woman. However, the cruel twist was the fact that his own wife had finally driven him with his belongings to the home of his new lover. Whilst this made me angry, it also revealed what I felt, i.e. that Mike would be within his rights to leave me and I should probably be that committed to him to participate in any breakdown as a willing player. All this is nonsense in the world of reason but emotions often rob us of the ability to act rationally; and what seems logical from the outside, may not prove so from the inside.

As for Mike, the discussions were to prove a trial in his willingness to face the situation for what it was. Coming to terms with childlessness was something that needed to be confronted and accepted for what it was. Avoidance strategies were to no avail. His inability to produce an answer from his extensive repertoire of abilities was to prove both threatening and character building. Strangely, in some ways, Mike never considered blaming me nor holding me responsible. As for me, I gained a great feeling of relief that the problem lay with my reproductive system and not with Mike's. I really did not want him to have to face a sense of personal inadequacy.

At all times, humour had provided a glorious means of keeping sanity amidst so many pressures. The final comment from our genial doctor as we had left his presence had been that we might try a variety of new positions for sexual intercourse—it might prove positively helpful.

Helpful or not, it provided us with a good deal of amusement—essential when the very act of love-making can be reduced to a mechanical attempt at conception, with all the pressures of childlessness finding an unwelcome focus around what should prove a relaxed and fun-filled time of expressing love and commitment to one another. We emerged from such exploits not with children but a new maxim which we offer to all married or prospective married couples. With regard to sexual intercourse, the said maxim runs as follows: 'As long as you break no bones, everything is permissible.' Of course, all maxims have a proviso and this is simply that both partners must be in agreement with all that is to take place in the marriage bed.

Chapter Four

'Hope has two beautiful daughters, courage and anger,' so claimed St Augustine. I had frequently encouraged myself with the oft repeated phrase 'new house, new baby'. Certainly, I looked to our move to Leeds with such eyes of hopeful anticipation. Hope was the mainspring of my life—hoping every time we made love that I would conceive. And then being wracked with disappointment with growing degrees of anger and bitterness at the start of my monthly period—my body's way of mocking my hopes of pregnancy. To live with this tension of 'am I, aren't I?' was exceptionally distressing and, in some ways, destructive. Yet as each new menstrual month began, Mike and I set our sights once more on the desired pregnancy and redoubled our efforts in that direction. As Mike has frequently said, he enjoys the practice! I too found it tremendously pleasurable.

It was just under two months when I received a letter granting me my first appointment at Leeds General Infirmary. The date was one when Mike was booked to be away from home. Rather than cancelling his engagement as he suggested, I gallantly insisted he go and that I would be fine attending the hospital on my own. Had I known then what I know now, I would never have been so apparently noble and strong. The whole issue of infertility is so closely woven into the fabric of one's emotions that every step of the way there are incredible peaks and troughs which produce laughter or tears at a moment's notice. I know I need my closest friend with me at such times of vulnerability—and my closest friend is Mike.

On the day itself Jane, a friend from the fellowship, came with me to the hospital, aptly titled the Hospital for Women, Outpatients Department. The waiting room was full of nervous ladies of all ages. The few, very few, men who had accompanied wife or girlfriend looked most incongruous and had the appearance of not belonging.

Summoned upstairs, I entered an examination room to be greeted by Mr Hancock, a gynaecologist. With the benefit of hindsight, I remain impressed with the attitude that prevailed throughout the hospital. This sought to ensure each patient felt as relaxed and remained as unembarrassed as possible. I was certainly treated with individual attention and made to feel that I remained as much a person as a patient.

Settled in the examination room, Mr Hancock

began by asking me a series of questions relating to my medical history—questions of a very general nature. He then enquired about my sex life, seeking to determine frequency (which in our case had much to do with Mike's travelling schedule) and level of pain, if any, during 'thrusting'. I was somewhat taken aback by the word 'thrusting' but this is the 'technical' language. Not simply technical but a very logical descriptive word. Recovering my composure, which had somewhat decomposed with the stark intimacy of such a word, I explained that I did suffer pain of varying degrees during penetration. Pain is always difficult to explain but the specialist continued to question me closely. It was a deep internal pain around the pelvic area was my more detailed description, quite pleased with my anatomical knowledge.

Throughout this interview, the statutory nurse took notes on my virgin file. The doctor then asked me to climb on to the examination couch for what proved a very thorough internal; more extensive than the usual GP's. At times this proved painful, the reason for which Mr Hancock explained having completed his investigations. He had identified inflamation of the pelvic region. The conclusion of this time was the suggestion that I return to the hospital for a brief two day visit for a minor operation, a laparoscopy. I was informed this simply entailed a small incision just below the belly button for the insertion of a laparoscope (a small telescope). This enables the specialist to take a close look at the reproductive organs. I readily agreed to this, descended the stairs, collected Jane from the waiting room and went to the desk in the entrance to arrange my hospitalization. The date was set for three weeks hence.

I was pleased that I was once again on course for a medical solution. Hope springs eternal and there was something happening, something to focus attention and expectations on. After all, pelvic inflamation did not sound too distressing. Later that day, as I waited for Mike to phone me, I sensed the first feeling of apprehension at what would be my first trip into hospital. I was grateful when the phone rang as it broke into my introspective reverie.

Mike's voice was cheery and he gave me his news before enquiring after my visit. I do find the phone a most distressing channel of communication. All the familiarity and warmth of a well-loved voice with none of the physical intimacy of its owner. Disembodied words however welcome always leave me with a sense of incompleteness and frustration. Amazed at my calmness, I reported the day's medical happenings, expressed my love for Mike, said goodbye, put down the phone and wept.

On his return a couple of days later, Mike took time to sit me down and say that if I didn't fancy a trip into hospital or wished to delay it, then he would fully support me and what's more make the necessary phone call to the hospital, etc. Throughout our childless pilgrimage, Mike has never urged or forced me to move at a pace faster than I felt comfortable with; nor has he insisted that I receive any treatment against my will. This has been very constructive since it has both allowed me to use Mike as a sounding board in thinking each issue through as it arose and allowed me to take each decision in my own right, assured of his total support once that decision is taken. There have been times when I've longed for Mike to take full responsibility—had he done so, however, I may well have blamed him in the low moments as I adjusted to some of the complicated consequences of infertility treatment of which at this stage I was blissfully ignorant.

DIARY

September 1982 What did they do at the hospital? Am experiencing phenomenal pain around my pelvic area—sex is a grit-your-teeth job now (sounds like an interesting position!). Mike very understanding. Is it that the hospital visit and my new information has made me more aware of the pain? The pain certainly appears to be very real and hurts, hurts, hurts.

September 1982 Woke last night with the most excruciating pain in my lower stomach. Thought I was about to die on the spot. However I lay, on my front, back, side, clutching pillow, the pain remained intense. Couldn't get back to sleep and began to sweat profusely. Mike slept on undisturbed in spite of my constant movement.

Night is not a good time to feel unwell. My mind had me sick with any number of terminal ailments as I turned and turned through the early hours. Eventually, frightened and alone, I woke Mike. Shook him fairly violently to break in upon his deep sleep, of which I was growing more and more jealous by the minute. Eventually, some sight of life as his eyes flickered open. 'Darling, darling,' I said with a fair degree of urgency. He grunted indicating he was awake. 'Mike, I'm dying, please call me an ambulance!' 'Darling, you're an ambulance,' he replied, before rolling over and going back to sleep. I was too stunned to know what to do. Tears rolled down my cheeks and, reverting to childhood, I comforted myself with the thought—when I'm dead in this bed in the morning, you'll be sorry! How I made it through the night, I don't know. I let Mike have it in the morning. 'Love is never having to say you're sorry,' he quipped! Too far, I thought, and all my anxiety and fear burst in two fast flowing rivers down either side of my face. We made up, Mike apologizing profusely, and all was well, apart from the fact that I retained a degree of anxiety about my pain, anxiety which I realized Mike also shared.

October 1982 The fateful day. My first trip to hospital. It was a Friday. Mike drove me across Leeds to the Hospital for Women proper. An older style building in a beautiful park-land setting. Appeared more like a retirement home than a hospital. Most appropriate, Mike said when I expressed this to him. I'm less anxious than I thought I would be. In fact, this is quite an adventure and I've quite a sense of anticipation.

On arrival, the booking in process begins—forms, blood tests and urine sample. All new to me and I obediently followed the nurses' orders. It's strange, the moment I arrived, all responsibility for my life has been lifted from my shoulders. All I've to do is follow the well-established routine. For my kind of character, this system is great. I'll just behave and seek to earn gold stars and come top of my ward. Surely if I'm good, there'll be no reason for anyone to hurt me!

Biggest shock so far! Nurse arrives to shave me prior to theatre. Something very intimate about pubic hair. I can't think why. Removed for fear of infection, I'm informed. Never mind, I simply yield to experience of the nurses. One thing, they are all so kind and courteous. Shaving followed by pre-med; my body enters a wonderful world in which it appears to be flying way above the ward. Also feel amazingly relaxed. Can one get pre-med injections from the chemist?

Porter arrives with trolley. Off to theatre we go—'play's good today,' he joked. I smiled unconcernedly. Into the anaesthetist's room for the general anaesthetic. 'Count to ten,' he said. 'One, two, three . . .' Next thing I knew, I was back in the ward. Tried sitting upright—aware of other patients mouthing something at me, head swimming deliciously, slight stabbing pain in stomach before falling backwards into a bed of pillows and a fitful sleep. Awake enough to talk with Mike during visiting. Slept well. Looking forward to being collected next day.

October 1982 Mike arrived at nine. I, having been awoken at 6.00 to follow hospital routine, had washed, eaten breakfast and then got dressed. Hospital empty and silent, or so it seemed. Gave me a Saturday feeling for which I was grateful—funny how each day of the week can be associated with a certain feeling and a different colour; well, in my mind's eye at least.

Romantic morning! Walked hand in hand with Mike down through the wooded driveway leading from the hospital and out on to the leaf strewn playing-fields beyond. Autumn dampness rose to refresh the nostrils, driving out the scent of sterilization. We talked little but I felt very close to Mike. Stopped off for coffee—no need for words. Smiled whenever we caught each other's eye. Sense of well-being, which neither of us wanted to drive away by starting a conversation.

It was to be a couple of weeks before I had to return to the Outpatients Department to get the results and comments on the laparoscopy. There was no more news until then and we both sensed a period free from the anxieties and tensions of our infertility and intended to enjoy it. Somehow no news was indeed good news and leaving everything in the hands of the doctors afforded us a brief oasis in the midst of our desert experience.

October 1982 One effect of the laparoscopy took me by surprise. In order to see more clearly, the doctor pumps air into the abdomen—or so I believe. Of course, what goes in must come out and I have been 'passing wind' at very regular intervals and extremely violently. Also slight ache in my shoulders—also caused from the air which finds its way around to different parts of the body. Not so much pain as discomfort. My outbursts provided a most suitable focus for humour —one which Mike took full advantage of!

COMMENTARY

These two weeks afforded us a much needed time of relaxation before entering into the next period of treatment. It was releasing to think our fate rested in the hands of the medical profession. We were hopeful of the results and so our optimism buoyed us up and we were extremely happy. I realized how far infertility had encroached on our life and lifestyle as we literally laughed and played during this time.

At the appointed time I returned to the Outpatients Department of the Hospital for Women. This occasion I ensured Mike was with me. We sat in the waiting-room—we are connoisseurs of waiting-rooms after years of experience. Mike leafed through innumerable women's magazines, pausing only to read the problem page. I'm convinced these are written solely for men, who seem to have an insatiable interest in them.

When I was summoned to visit the specialist,

Mike rose, crossed the room with me but was prevented from ascending the stairs by a nurse. 'But this is my wife,' he protested, to no avail. He was despatched back to the waiting room and still more problem pages.

It does seem strange that I should be able to bare all to innumerable doctors and medical students but my own husband, who is quite used to seeing his own wife naked, must be excluded. The expectant mother entering labour is afforded the comfort and assurance of her husband in the delivery room and yet the woman in the trauma of infertility treatment is robbed of her closest confidant at a time of severe emotional upheaval. I'm told that it's because husbands may get upset seeing strange men in white coats investigating their wife—but there again they may not. Nothing can be less sexually arousing than lying half undressed on an examination table, one's mind concentrating on resisting the temptation to tense up before the anticipated internal, as well as anxious over what medical pronouncement will flow from the specialist's lips. To have one's husband by the hand and be able to gaze into his face would be a very pleasant experience and encouragement.

However, this was not to be and I found myself listening intently to all Mr Hancock said. A further reason I had wanted Mike there was that he remembers facts and details a lot more clearly than I do and to have had his ears in on the discussions would have proved useful.

The result of the laparoscopy had revealed that

I have extensive endometriosis. This affected both my Fallopian tubes, both my ovaries, and my uterus. It was suggested I enter hospital for major surgery, during which the specialist would use a laser to clear all the endometriosis out of the system, thus enabling the tubes to collect the eggs from the ovaries, carrying them to make contact with the sperm and hence become impregnated. At which point I would have conceived and a child would have been created.

I asked Mr Hancock what 'major surgery' meant in practical terms. He explained patiently that they would make a large incision along my bikini line (similar to an hysterectomy cut) and take the time necessary to clear the system. I would be in hospital for around ten days and would require a period of recovery at home afterwards. Obviously, I agreed to this course of action on the grounds that it offered me the chance of children. However, I was disappointed that the investigative surgery had not provided a simpler solution to our dilemma. I returned to Mike in the waiting-room to bring him up to date with developments, while one of Mr Hancock's team, a jovial German doctor, went to look at the operating schedules in order to give me a date.

Mike was just assimilating the information I'd brought him when we were summoned to the front desk and offered a date just three weeks hence. We were taken aback at the closeness of the date but readily agreed. Leaving, all we talked about was cancelling our planned trip to visit my sister in Australia, arranged for Christmas. This was a disappointment and one I felt keenly, having been very close to Alison whilst growing up, but the desire to be pregnant was certainly my overriding concern. We toyed briefly with the idea of risking Australia anyway, trusting I would be up to it. In the event it was just as well we cancelled.

Mike was especially attentive over this period. He re-arranged his diary so that he would be able to care for me on my return from hospital. Fortunately, it ran into Christmas, a time when Mike always takes an extended holiday.

Facing a trip into hospital, I suddenly realized I had no nightdresses, dressing gown, etc. We therefore went on an extended shopping trip on which we selected suitable night attire. Not used to spending so much money at any one time, I constantly tried to curb Mike's extravagance. He insisted on selecting and buying me a beautiful dressing gown; this was followed by a wash bag, flannels, sweet-smelling soap, new toothbrush, and a variety of other 'toys'. In fact, my hospitalization was turning into quite an occasion.

As the day drew nearer, my prayer intensified significantly—I was going to say improved but I think intensified better describes it. Mid-week prior to my departure, the fellowship gathered round me to pray. I felt something of a celebrity —it was most agreeable to be the focus of so much attention. I smiled as someone prayed with great sincerity that, whilst on the operating table, the Lord would 'undertake' for me. I knew what they meant but I saw the funny side.

Not only did the church rally round, but my mother travelled up from London to spend a day with me—something I found very touching and of which I was deeply appreciative. No matter how old one gets, there is always something reassuring about having one's mother there. Love and concern appeared to be surrounding me on all sides. It gave a tremendous boost and I was most grateful.

I was due to be admitted on Wednesday morning at 9.30 a.m. We arrived at around 9.15 a.m. and were shown to the waiting-room just at the end of the ward. The girl whose bed I was to take was waiting for her boyfriend to come and pick her up. We chatted briefly and I discovered that she had had an ovary removed. She was obviously still alive and looked fit and well, so the surgeons must know their business—I should survive my visit!

Once my bed was ready, I was asked to change into my nightdress. Strange having been dressed for so short a time and not feeling the slightest bit unwell. A wardrobe was supplied next to my bed for my clothes, something I found encouraging because I felt I could get up and leave the moment that things got out of hand. Strange the way our minds work in such situations. Mike had left, promising to visit me that evening.

In bed and the nurse visited to run through the booking-in procedure with which I was to become so familiar. Urine sample, blood pressure, a few questions and answers. The day passed slowly. Lunch time eventually arrived and all able-bodied patients made their way to the dining-room. I chatted to several of the ladies and extended my medical knowledge a fair degree. Even though I had magazines to read, letters to write, etc, by 4.00 p.m. I was bored! I found the telephone and rang Mike. Informing him of my predicament, he told me to enjoy my idleness and fitness, to get some good rest and prepare for the operation. Visiting time could not come soon enough.

Once it arrived, I was thrilled to catch sight of Mike's familiar figure strolling up the ward. I realized for the first time how important it was for folk in hospital to receive visitors, and I'd only been in the ward for around ten hours! As he got to my bed, Mike opened his jacket to reveal flowers, sweets and fruit—and I wasn't even ill. Sitting himself down, I heard all about the shopping, washing and cleaning—role reversal *par excellence*. It also revealed how hard it was to sustain an interesting conversation for the one and a half hours of visiting time. When does one sit down with husband or wife and talk for such a length of time? I couldn't believe we ran out of conversation. I'd have liked a good cuddle but it didn't seem an appropriate setting.

Before he left, Mike and I prayed together and then agreed that for future visiting times, he would bring in board games to fill the time and give us a focus for our time together.

Mike left and following a late-night drink, lights were turned out at 10.00 p.m. and I easily drifted off to sleep. I didn't realize it was not so easy for Mike. He found the house very empty without me and couldn't get around to going to bed. As I slept, Mike was prowling around our home, listening to the radio, flicking through the TV channels, dipping into books and feeling somewhat aimless, there being no way he could influence my situation. He apparently went to bed around 2.00 a.m. for a very disturbed night's sleep.

Chapter Five

Abortion. A word guaranteed to create an immediate reaction of one sort or another. The Oxford English Dictionary defines abortion as 'the procuring of premature delivery so as to destroy offspring' or 'Arrest of development of any organ'. Basically, the interference of some external force to interrupt natural growth and development. As a Christian, I had over a number of years come to accept that life begins at conception. This made abortion a crime against humanity since it destroyed a human life. Obviously, many are the arguments ranged against such a position, often based on hypothetical situations. Unfortunately, although very painful, real life tragedies occur and we should not build a moral position on exceptional circumstances. We need to discover the moral principle at the centre of the argument—in the case of recognition of a living God, it is God himself—and then sensitively apply that to each and every case as it arises. Principles are essential for establishing an absolute moral framework but the essence of life is in meeting real people enduring real pain and interpreting such principles in ways that enable them to see the absolute behind the moral framework—that is God himself.

Life is lived in society where people rub shoulders with people; individuals suffer tragedy which by various means and media, we are all invited to participate in to some degree (for example, the Hungerford massacre or the Zeebrugge disaster) and our heart goes out to such individuals. Is it kindest to seek immediately to ameliorate what we perceive to be their greatest tragedy or should we rather assist them over a period of time to focus their eyes on their life, their place and future in society and provide a point of meeting for them with God himself? We all live our lives according to one code or another. The Christian world view is to my mind the ultimate world view. A God who cared for a lost and hurting humanity to the degree that he took upon himself human flesh, lived as man amongst men to reveal the nature of God and the nature and possibility of relationship with God, is a God to whom I gladly offer worship and service, for as Noel Richards has so potently written in one of his songs: 'You're the only one who died for me'—and so he is. A mighty God determined to win the world to himself puts himself on Death Row and suffers execution unjustly for me. I know of no

philosopher, religious leader, intellectual thinker
—and heaven knows, there are any number to
choose from—who proved so committed to the
welfare of humanity that he got his own hands
dirty to sort the situation out.

The magic of the whole picture is that Jesus—
God in human form—rose from the dead; as a
historian, this has never failed to leave a great
impression on me. The circumstantial evidence
for the resurrection is overwhelming and I know
of no other religious leader who ever predicted he
would rise from the dead or who contemporary
historians recorded had risen from the dead. To
dismiss an absolute moral code based upon
Christian principles is one thing, but to dismiss
the absolute, God himself, who gave rise to and
supplies reason for such a moral code is quite
another. And to do so unthinkingly as so many do
is, to say the least, criminal.

As I lay in hospital, I began to realize by various
comments and through a number of conversations that abortions were being carried out on
this ward. It came as a bolt out of the blue and I
found myself totally unprepared for this news. As
I lay waiting for an operation which would, I
hoped, enable me to produce a new life, there
were those following me into theatre terminating
life. What a topsy-turvy world! I was to discover
that in every gynaecological ward there was this
apparent confusion of interests. Some women
sought terminations, others (younger than myself) were in for sterilization, unable to stop themselves conceiving, while still others, like myself,

were drawing upon the skill of the medics to give them the opportunity of bearing children.

I directed no particular animosity against those in the first two categories but did feel that the Health Service might have proved a little more subtle. At a time of extreme emotional instability, here I was confronted with the destruction of the very life I yearned for. So often when expressing my position on abortion, I had been accused of being heartless and unfeeling. How I longed for someone to feel with me now in my vulnerability and isolation—an infertile woman who counted expended foetuses to send her off to sleep!

Perhaps the most galling of all such situations occurred some years later when I was a patient at a London hospital. I was booked for a further laparoscopy and had been told to report to the ward at 9.30 a.m. When we arrived, Mike dutifully carrying my overnight bag, the ward had big no-entry signs up with directions to press the bell button for attention. The button was solidly taped up so that it was immovable. Mike attracted the attention of an auxiliary nurse and pointed out our predicament. She disappeared into the ward and next moment, two eyes appeared around the door, the rest of the lady's face being covered by an operating mask. I said I had come to register, she suggested we go and get a meal. Mike pointed out it was only 9.30 a.m. and that we had only just had breakfast. Taken aback, she thought for a moment before promising to find someone to attend to me. We were told to sit down outside the ward in the corridor. At this point, Mike urged me to quit and come home—I insisted on going through with it all, something I was later to consider as a wrong decision.

Anyhow, eventually I was given a bed on the ward and discovered the reason for my non-admittance earlier in the day. A small area at the end of the ward had been screened off to provide a make-shift operating theatre and a number of abortions were then carried out. I could have cried: for myself; for the lost lives; for the women involved. I didn't, perhaps I should have. What a confused world we live in. The NHS has given a whole new meaning to the word 'care'.

Returning to Leeds, amongst the other women were those in for hysterectomies, bladder repairs and general gynaecological treatment. The ward was a very friendly ward.

DIARY

October 1982 Thursday dawned. Operation day minus one. 6.00 a.m. does not seem so dreadfully early in hospital. The business of the routine is helpful. Strange having washed and eaten breakfast not to have to get dressed. Wander to day-room while ward is cleaned.

Summoned back to my bed for doctor's rounds. Shaved once again; still found it an unpleasant experience to which to adjust. Mr Hancock arrived, only to ask me to attend the examination-room at 3.00 that afternoon. I agreed—not that I think I had any real choice in the matter. He then asked if I minded a few student observers being present at my examination. Convinced everyone must be given as much encouragement in learning their craft as possible, I nodded my assent. And then he was gone, a blur of white surrounded by an entourage of white coats and grey nurses' uniforms.

The examination-room lay at the heart of an intricate web of corridors. I was taken there by a nurse. Great, all my thinking is done for me in this place. No sooner had I clambered on to the couch and prepared myself for the umpteenth examination, than the door opened and in walked Mr Hancock followed by one, two, three, four . . . eleven young, some very handsome, male medical students—and . . . one lady. I felt somewhat at a disadvantage, and no one to introduce us!

During my examination—longer than on previous occasions—I learnt from this assembled group of medics that I didn't have cancer and that my general health was excellent. I was grateful for such encouragements. I'm sure my predicament provided an invaluable milestone in these young doctors' training but some greater measure of warning would have helped me prepare myself a little better for it. Flat on a bed, legs akimbo, and naked is not my accustomed fashion of greeting gentlemen I have not had the privilege of meeting before. For the first time, I felt rather like a slab of meat, a feeling that was heightened as the specialist posed questions about my condition to different students as if I were no more than a textbook diagram.

While I was in this state of vulnerability Mr Hancock ended the examination by informing me, very gently I must add, that he might need to remove my left Fallopian tube and left ovary during the operation, since it was so badly affected by endometriosis. I returned to the ward shell-shocked and lay on my bed thinking.

If they removed a tube, would I still be normal? Could I reproduce? Would I need to take drugs to balance all my hormones? I suddenly realized how ignorant I was—fell asleep with all these anxious thoughts buzzing around in my head.

Evening time and Mike's visit—none too soon. Nervous now as the operation seemed much more real the closer it got. Mike did well keeping the conversation light. Asking him a pile of irrelevant questions—was he eating properly? What about his washing? And his ironing? Said he was OK since appointing two Swedish au pairs! Prayed together—hard letting him go. Felt I was on my own. Took sleeping tablet as advised by the nurses. Slept very soundly.

November 1982 Woken by tea trolley trundling along ward. Today is the day. Big notice on bed reads, 'Nil by Mouth'. Sacrifice giving up my early morning cuppa.

Directed to shower; used non-perfumed soap and told not to put on any talcum powder. Returned to my bed to find barrier gown and 'J' cloth style head-dress awaiting me. Put on the gown and talked with other patients similarly clad who were due in theatre that day. Much fear

88

evident. People are very honest and friendly when frightened. I found myself quietly praying for these women—nothing very noble, just happened quite naturally. A number of folk commented on my serene approach to the forthcoming ordeal. I was glad something of Jesus shone through in this situation.

Approached by nurse to be told of batting order for the day. I was second on the list. My expected time of departure for theatre was 10.30 a.m.; pre-med due at 9.00 a.m. I was told to be in bed by then. I was. Pre-med duly given and I settled back expecting to fly as before. My rest was soon interrupted by the arrival of the porter with canvas stretcher and poles. 'Too soon,' I said. 'Wrong person'—fearing I might emerge minus a leg in a case of mistaken identity. Patiently, it was pointed out that the first patient was unable to go to theatre, so everyone was being brought forward. Crawling on to the stretcher, I shut my eyes and settled down for my trip into oblivion.

It took some time to get to theatre. An endless round of checking began. My name, my ward, my date of birth. I kept being asked if I was Kathleen Morris. 'Yes,' I replied repeatedly. Next hurdle: lift out of order. I was pushed down ramps and corridors on what appeared an interminable journey. At one stage we left the cover and warmth of the hospital buildings and went out into the sharp November air. I felt somewhat indignant at this. Headline flashed across my mind: 'Woman enters hospital with infertility, leaves with pneumonia.'

Eventually, reach anaesthetist's room—checks name, age, ward once again before sending me to sleep with a tiny prick in the arm and the sound of counting numbers in my ears.

COMMENTARY

My knowledge of operating theatres is nil. Only what I have glimpsed on films. This trip revealed no more of their secrets. The very next thing I remember is being gently tapped and my name, 'Kathleen, Kathleen,' being repeated by a nurse seeking some reaction as I lay in the recovery-room. Once my eyes were open and sufficient reaction had been gauged, I was wheeled back to the ward—whether by lift or by corridor I do not recollect.

I learnt later that I had actually been in theatre for around two hours, which from all accounts is a long time to be anaesthetized.

In the ward again I remember little save snatches of incidents in the first few hours. My eyesight was blurred. My blood pressure, pulse and temperature were taken several times. Once I asked for a drink of water, my mouth feeling so dry and parched. This is normal with a general anaesthetic. The nurse only allowed me a sip but once she turned her back, I gulped several mouthfuls and was immediately sick. I only sipped after that. I also asked what time it was (the most frequently asked question by patients returning from theatre)—it was 1.30 p.m. At some point I was told Mike had phoned and had been told I was safely back from theatre, also my mother. I slept a lot—a strange business of drifting in and out of consciousness with no sense of time passing or any awareness of bandages, wounds and other paraphernalia to aid the recovering patient.

Dinner arrived. I was encouraged to eat a little. Did so. A very little. At 6.30 p.m. the doctor arrived to inform me that they had successfully cleared both tubes and ovaries, and hence nothing had been removed. In my stupor I'm sure I was not as ecstatic as I should have been but thanked the doctor as best I could. He was evidently quite excited at the success of the operation, which I found encouraging. It was also very sweet of him to ensure he told me so soon, especially before Mike visited that evening.

I continued to drift in and out of sleep, one time when I woke, Mike was there, holding my hand. I tried to sit up and talk to him but immediately collapsed, exhausted, back on to the bed. For the first time, I became aware of the drip in my arm—this was very restricting, mostly because of terrible visions of my inadvertently ripping it out of my arm. This I must say would be virtually impossible. I gathered my thoughts and, concentrating all my energy, informed Mike of the good news about saving tube and ovary. This task completed, I continued to drift in and out of consciousness. I don't recall him leaving.

Next morning, I awoke feeling very much better. I was fully conscious now and aware of the drip in my arm and a drain attached to my wound carrying blood away to a small plastic bag. At this stage I was confined to bed and remember well the struggles with bed pans and commodes. I was excited with the news the surgeon had brought me. The day was Saturday. Afternoon visiting and I couldn't wait to see Mike. One difficulty I did find was eating. My appetite had totally disappeared. In fact, I only picked at food for several days until eventually Mike ordered me to eat something substantial. Shocked by the seriousness of his manner, I did force myself to consume more than I wanted and only learnt after leaving hospital of the concern the nursing staff had expressed to Mike about my eating pattern, the reason for his heavy-handed approach.

DIARY

December 1982 3.00 p.m. and Mike arrived. I am impressed he is never late. More chocolate, flowers, etc. What a boy! Wide awake, I jabbered on non-stop. I requested the loo. The nurse instructed Mike to help me along the corridor to the WC. First time on my feet since operation. Progress was slow and somewhat ridiculous. I refused to stand upright, frightened I'd burst my wound. What's more, I could only shuffle my feet along the floor. This was my impersonation of the Hunchback of Notre Dame! Not only did I have to take myself to the loo, but I also had to push my drip along on its castors and carry my drainbag as a kind of Dorothy luggage. It took a good ten minutes to reach the loo and an equal amount of time to ensconse myself on it. Mike was very attentive but obviously a bit ham-fisted.

Having been to the loo, I then had to wash my undercarriage on the bidet before shuffling back to bed. I collapsed gratefully on my mattress, exhausted and committed to never going to the loo again.

Talked excitedly about starting a family. I was convinced it was all plain sailing from now on in. I could not contain my excitement. Laughter was easy and a great weight appeared to have been removed from my mind. All I wanted was to leave hospital and become pregnant.

COMMENTARY

I was in hospital for a week after the operation, getting better by the day. Mike allowed friends to visit as he saw my strength return—visiting time did exhaust me but remained a very precious part of my daily routine. This was a time for making friends with other patients. Being gregarious, I enjoyed this and I found ample opportunity to talk about my love for and friendship with God.

One lovely incident stands out. Opposite me, an elderly nun was receiving treatment for cancer. I found it very humbling to be invited to pray for her and was touched by her gratitude. All I'd done was pray. Her graciousness and peace in the face of a lot of physical pain and not a very hopeful diagnosis was striking. It was much more than skin deep—she really was at rest at the very core of her being; what a fine testimony. Mike and I prayed regularly for Sister Joan and we were encouraged by her.

The only problem came when it was time for changing my first dressing. When the nurse arrived and informed me, I instantly burst into tears and begged her, literally begged her, to postpone it to the next day. I had only ever witnessed one dressing change. This was when Mike had the first dressing removed from his big toe which had had the nail removed. On that occasion I had had to apologize, while rising from my seat, and leave the room. And it wasn't even my toe! I took some convincing before letting the nurse near my stomach, and I am so grateful for her patience. Needless to say, it hurt not a bit—I did feel silly!

Thoughout this period, I was given pain-killers. I shall never know if I needed them or not, for I never suffered a moment of pain during my whole stay. All I had to do was concentrate on getting stronger. This task seemed easier once the drain and the drip were removed.

Chapter Six

It was very exciting news when the doctor informed me that my left Fallopian tube and ovary were still with me and had been cleared of endometriosis. While I slept off the anaesthetic, Mike had returned home from the hospital beside himself with joy and praising God. Throughout our pilgrimage of infertility, we had prayed; sometimes fairly generally, at other times very specifically. Just before entering hospital, with the endometriosis diagnosis fresh in our minds, Mike had spent a lot of time praying for me. As he prayed, he saw very clearly in his mind's eye a picture of what he took to be my ovaries and tubes clearing of all obstruction. He was absolutely convinced that everything was cleared—as convinced as I've seen him of anything. With the news that I might lose an ovary and tube, he remained convinced that this would not in fact occur. He didn't make an issue of it before the operation, knowing that I would in some ways feel a failure, worrying about both the operation and the possible loss of part of my reproductive system and what that would do to Mike's faith. In fact, I know I would not have seen Mike's faith as misplaced but rather taken the blame myself—quite irrationally.

Hence, with the news that all had been cleared, Mike was worship-weary by the time he crawled into bed. Interestingly enough, when at a later date I was referred to the endometriosis specialist at Kings College Hospital on the assumption that my earlier endometriosis had recurred (we were informed at Leeds that it was regenerative), Mike remained totally certain that it hadn't. A further laparoscopy proved Mike's confidence to be well founded and left the medics in some ways dumb-founded. There was not one trace of endo-metriosis to be found anywhere in my body. When God speaks clearly to us, we can certainly place full confidence in all that he says.

Obviously, an issue like childlessness does drive one to ask certain questions of God. Once we discovered we were to experience difficulties with conceiving, we immediately turned to prayer. These were prayers arising from a very selfish motivation. Initially, we felt it could only be a test from God and as soon as we became a little more spiritual, hey presto, I'd become pregnant. This was not to be the case. However, we did learn a number of significant lessons.

It soon became evident that our childlessness put us in a place in which God had our undivided attention. We were desperate to hear what he had to say about children—only as we spent time together with him, he appeared to have nothing to say on the subject. There were all sorts of other areas—attitudes, priorities, relationships—that he spoke very directly to us about, but little on children. Obediently, we responded to all that we heard but felt increasingly desperate for children.

We also grasped at straws. Any scripture we turned up we tended to interpret in terms of our childlessness. I remember turning up Isaiah 40: 1–2 one day: 'Comfort, comfort my people, says your God. Speak tenderly to Jerusalem, and proclaim to her that her hard service has been completed, that her sin has been paid for, that she has received from the Lord's hand double for all her sins.' I immediately assumed my childlessness was 'hard service'. We had always wanted twins hence 'double' here meant two babies not one. Through conferences and from the preaching we had recently heard, we were very aware of the *rhema* or specific word of God. This was surely the *rhema* word. And it wasn't a single instance; I came across many other such *rhema* words over the months. All we did was thank God and hold fast to these words. However, our conviction in them, our confidence, ebbed away as the months continued to pass without the slightest bulge to show for them. To this day, we both have a measure of confusion over these 'words'. Should we hold fast to them? Reject them? Are we wrong to hold them? It is amazing the theological gymnastics we will perform when we are in need and

God is our only resource.

Not only were there words we found but as more folk discovered our predicament, well-meaning Christians brought words to us. Many of these, in retrospect, came with love and affection but were no more than the compassionate, caring aspirations of fellow Christian pilgrims trying to make some sense of God in the midst of life's realities. They wanted us to have children; they hoped we would; they verbalized their hopes.

Another group of people, however, took it upon themselves to identify areas of sin in our lives—wrong attitudes, rampant demons and worse—which blocked God's blessing. The major problem here was that few hung around long enough to guide us from these murky depths that might obstruct conception. And none wanted to risk their reputation in their revelation by forth-rightly declaring the nature of the blockage, deal-ing with it and standing by us until we conceived. The church seems filled at times with bearers of bad tidings, whose rate of creative productivity within the kingdom is nil. I hope God throws them all out—they will be a bore in heaven, an eternal bore!

We did receive counsel and prophetic words from senior churchmen and we hold to these still. All saw us with children, indeed a number prophesied twins without knowing our desire for them. To date, we remain childless but we will hold fast to these promises. In doing so clouds of doubt often obscure the promise and it would be ridiculous to deny the doubts. Yet even when shrouded with doubt, we keep our eyes upon the peak of promise, although obscured from view. We know it will come back in focus again and spur us on. In fact, as Mike has said so often, he will go to his death-bed believing God's promise of children, because if you can't trust God, who can you trust?

I found it very refreshing to be honest about my doubts. Initially, neither of us dared mention that our prayers might not be answered. We were trapped into the heresy of confusing the power of positive thinking with faith. However, as time passed, we both found it possible to consider, 'What if we didn't have a family?' Initially, we felt very naughty even talking in such terms but we needed to talk it all through. I found it a tremendous pressure valve to be free to express my doubts and uncertainties. We did find it hard with so many well-meaning Christians praying very earnestly—and usually very loudly!—for us. We felt a kind of guilt or betrayal of their intensity. But it was a firm foundation for living. Our desperation for a family was such that we instituted virtually all advice we were given. We were encouraged to get children to pray that we might have a family—we were grateful for the way Rob and Marion White's daughters took up the task of praying. On one occasion when we were staying with them in Banstead, we joined together for family prayers. The twins prayed aloud and with great passion, that God would give us the children we longed for. We retired to bed. The next morning we were awoken by the twins knocking on the bedroom door, bringing us an early morning cup of tea. Inviting them to enter, I fixed my eyes on them and dared them to ask if I was pregnant yet. I could sense them checking me out to see if there was an air of pregnancy about me.

The White twins have been very faithful in praying for us. I remember giving them a lift home from a staff conference one time. As we approached the Blackwall Tunnel, Jo asked, 'Do you want to have a family, Katey?' I replied in the affirmative. After a moment's pause she said, 'You do know what to do, don't you?' Once again, I said that I believed I did. No sooner had I finished than she added, 'It's called making love, you know.' Mike, who was driving, nearly left the road and I decided it was better to let the conversation drop at this point. The lovely thing about children is their honesty and their ability to keep faith with God, even though prayers go apparently unanswered. The White girls were a great encouragement to us.

We also presented ourselves for ministry at every available opportunity. If there was a spiritual obstruction, we wanted it shifted—and fast! In retrospect, I believe we may well have been a little naïve in all this. I've lost count of both the number of people who prayed for me and the variety of issues 'ministered' to. Many also directed their attention to my 'sharp tongue', 'harsh character', 'sarcasm', 'cynicism', 'self-deprecation', etc. I constantly tried to re-order my lifestyle in line with the latest 'input' I received. Mike was also 'ministered' to along similar lines. Unfortunately, the longer this went on—and we are talking about years—without the glimmer of a pregnancy, the less enthusiasm there was, confidence declined and depression set in. Depression not simply about remaining childless but that we might perhaps be beyond the reach of God himself. When Mike expressed this, self-pity was identified as the problem. We retreated from the main forum populated by Christian activists eagerly waiting to clap hands on anyone in need.

Some of the teaching relating to childlessness we took very seriously. We prayed this through ourselves and invited those we loved and trusted to pray for us. These areas included hereditary contact with the Masonic movement and involvement with the occult, either personally or by other family members back through the generations. Mike had also often joked that we would be childless from early years of marriage and he felt obliged to acknowledge a deep-seated fear he had carried over a number of years. All this may sound far-fetched—and perhaps it is. We still do not have children, have not even conceived, so the value of such ministry in the cold light of day may remain questionable. However, these were areas in which we felt very happy to receive ministry once the scriptural basis had been explained to us. There is a point, however, where one cannot face publicly identifying one's need and hence inviting ministry. We were also saddened and tired by the forthright confidence of those who ministered—it would have been great for someone to say, 'This might not work'; also we felt a number of people put the responsibility for the success of the ministry back on to us, a burden which would have proved intolerable had we not together agreed to refuse to accept it. Finally, there were those we invited to pray but who from that point onwards, never enquired as to how things were going in the light of their prayers and ministry, and who also made it quite clear that they were not especially keen to talk about the subject should we air it.

Our prayer life together was good and constructive. I found I could weep before God and it was refreshing. Mike learnt that he could let me without feeling compelled to 'minister' to me. He also discovered that there were times to offer me affection and hug me, while at others, it was best to leave me to sob quietly, prayerfully with God alone. Raw emotion is a very strange human characteristic. I realize how little room the church allows for emotional expression, which at times is essential for healing and a manifestation of the heart of God. Mike also learnt to cry through this period. This helped him to express the indignation and pain he felt on a wider front too, for powerless people worldwide.

Of course, there were occasions when my tears turned in upon themselves and spoke more of self-pity than concern for our childless state. As we recognized this, I gave Mike full permission to seek to point this out to me and draw me away from my selfish introspection. Self-pity was my most unhealthy and yet ever-present emotion. I stress that I gave Mike permission to seek to get a grip of me because often I would resist his approaches, not wanting to lay aside my 'poor me' syndrome. We concluded he would have to leave me to it in such circumstances, since I alone held the keys to my own freedom and there was nothing he could do to help me, apart from identifying my attitude and encouraging, cajoling, bullying me to shake it off. If I didn't want to, I wouldn't. I was totally responsible for my own condition.

As we argued with, railed against, cried out to and wept before God, we discovered the reality of a relationship with him and with each other. We had to learn how to handle each other—sometimes we failed disastrously. Shouting at each other, ignoring each other, staring out each other. At other times we made contact with each other at a very deep level: cuddling, taking a walk hand in hand, lying in bed talking our way through the early hours of the morning. Our respect for each other grew, our love deepened, our dependence was total. Had we not found one another at the heart of our problem, we would not have made it through the extreme times of pain. We so appreciated the fact that God had given us to each other to love and care for each other. Our relationship with God grew. We realized we really did love him. We chat to him every moment of the day with great familiarity, for we really do sense we know him as a dear friend and constant companion. Words by themselves are incapable of communicating the nature and reality of a relationship with God. What is required is a personal encounter—regularly. One benefit of our childlessness has been a deepening sense of the reality of God himself and growing sense of commitment to him over and above everyone and everything else.

Of the conclusions we drew, the following proved the most vital. As a married couple, we do not have a divine right to children; nor does any married couple. This perspective is increasingly hard to sustain in the light of recent developments in medical techniques offering test-tube babies. It appears the whole technology is marketed on the basis that childlessness is the worst possible calamity to affect a couple. This is probably untrue. I believe situations where one partner has multiple sclerosis, or cancer are far worse. Infertility is not a disease. In an age and society where we expect to have whatever we want, there is tremendous popular pressure for pumping vast amounts of money into research in In Vitro techniques, so that people may have what they want. Any couple has the capacity to come to terms with their infertility and learn to live within the constraints that places upon them, while exploring the horizons and fields of opportunity it opens up to them.

In considering the book of Job in the Old Testament, we discovered God was in fact sovereign. I'm sure Job did not choose to lose his family, his livelihood and his health but lose them he did. Eventually, having proved his faithfulness, God restored everything—he was twice as prosperous as originally and also had a new family. And there's the rub; a new family. He will still have carried the pain of the original loss; not altogether the totally happy ending everyone normally speaks of. We were to learn that God places us here on the earth for the brief span which is our natural life to live for his glory. Nothing more, nothing less.

Mike travelled to Russia in October 1986 to visit Valeri Barinov, the Christian rock musician, on behalf of Jubilee Campaign. He was struck by the way Valeri constantly stressed that he only wanted 'to live for Jesus' glory'. This, having had all his ribs broken, been drenched in freezing cold water, locked in solitary confinement, suffering physical as well as great psychological torture. What's more, when Mike pointed out that if he were to tell Valeri's story publicly in the West, then it may be treated as a provocative act by the Soviet government and send Valeri back to prison, separated once again from his family and subject him to further physical and mental abuse, his immediate response (and Mike put it to him on three separate occasions) was that if God wanted him back in a labour camp, he would go. He was convinced he only wanted to live for Jesus' glory. Childlessness has served to remind us that as slaves of Christ, we lay aside all our personal rights; belonging to Christ, we live to glorify him alone: he calls the shots; he is the boss; Jesus Christ is Lord. As it has so often been said, 'If he is not Lord of all, he is not Lord at all.'

Throughout our childless journey, the place of prayer has been an important one in focusing our attention on the God we love and serve. It is true to say we have asked the question 'Why us?'; we have got angry, depressed, been filled with self-pity and been exceptionally negative. However, our faith has been increased not decreased; our love and commitment developed, not diminished. It is our constant prayer that we have the children we pray for and ache for. However, as we pray, we are aware that the moment I become pregnant, life will change very radically. No doubt I'll have something to say about that too!

Chapter Seven

Whether we be young or old,
Our destiny, our being's heart and home,
Is with infinitude, and only there;
With hope it is, hope that can never die,
Effort, and expectation, and desire,
And something evermore about to be.

So wrote Wordsworth. As I completed my week of recovery in hospital, hope was at a very high level. I dreamed often and only of children. I allowed my mind to range over forbidden territory: prams, buggies, baby clothes; the joy of telling parents they would be grandparents. To this day I'm not sure if some of the anaesthetic had not got lodged in my system, for I was so 'high'!

The day I was due to be discharged, Mr Hancock made his rounds and stopped by my bed to wish me well and discuss further treatment, explaining my tubes, ovaries and uterus were now 'cleared out' and that conceiving should no longer prove a problem. A tremor of excitement ran through my body. He went on to explain that endometriosis was known to be regenerative and that he would recommend that we put my body through a false pregnancy. This could be achieved by placing me on the contraceptive Pill for nine months.

'He who has never hoped can never despair'—this produced the second hysterical outburst of my stay in the Leeds General Infirmary. Nine months hence seemed light years away. I wanted to be pregnant now, now, now! Didn't anybody understand? Mr Hancock continued to explain that gynaecological surgery left the patient highly emotional—wasn't I the living proof!—and tearful. He wouldn't insist I took the Pill but highly recommended it. I for my part felt considerably better at the thought of avoiding this proposed treatment.

Time to leave hospital and Mike was at the other end of the country. He was training BYFC team members in Norfolk. The most attentive one of his audience was our dog, Dileas, whom he had had to take with him rather than leave at home for his visit. It would not be until mid-evening that he would arrive back in Leeds. Had I realized the weather conditions he drove through, I would have worried for him every mile of the way. He only left the road once—thick fog obliterating a sharp bend. Fortunately, no damage was done to car and driver.

I had had to dress and pack mid-afternoon so

that my bed could be prepared for its next occupant. At 9.00 p.m. Mike burst into the hospital to find me sitting in the waiting area at the end of the ward. He was given strict instructions by the staff nurse that I was to do nothing, not even make a cup of tea. I had been undergoing some physio to get me using my stomach again but was under orders not to lift anything. Once told, I didn't want to for fear of ripping my wound wide open.

Since I was used to the warmth of the ward, Mike insisted on my wrapping up very well against the elements. To be honest, I found his insistence somewhat trying but let him wind scarves around me and button my coat from top to bottom. All I wanted was to be away, to return to my home and, surprisingly maybe, see my dog again. I stepped out of the hospital doors into the night, supported by Mike's arm. The cold hit me— it was like walking into a brick wall. All my strength seemed to drain away. I clung tightly to Mike as he steered me across the car park to my carriage. I asked for the heaters to be put on full blast.

I shall never forget the joy of getting home. It has always been a source of great enjoyment to me, whether visiting friends or on holiday, to return home. There is something warm, familiar, secure about one's house. Ten days in hospital and I was thrilled to be back where I belonged. I sat in the lounge reading letters. Circulars, anything that made me feel 'normal' after the routine of hospital life. Mike made me a cup of tea before suggesting I retire. I needed no prompting but unfortunately, bed meant climbing the stairs. Five minutes it took to ascend those thirteen stairs. At the top I felt totally washed out—as if I'd completed a marathon. It was the last time I attempted those stairs for the next five days.

The change from hospital to home had quite an impact upon me physically. Before leaving the ward, I felt I was just about fit once again. The journey home, the cold (we never seemed to be able to heat our home to the same temperature as the ward), the lack of routine all conspired to exhaust me. I realized just how major an effect surgery had had on me. Mike had to do everything, which he did very well. Initially, this was a treat, but I soon wanted to be up and about but was incapacitated. Being by nature an activist, I found this period of enforced rest quite a trial by the end of just a few days. Convalescence may have aided my bodily, physical recovery but mentally and emotionally it made me short-tempered and not the nicest person to know. I was grateful for the many visitors I received; they became my ears and eyes in a world of hustle and bustle from which I was temporarily excluded.

The joy of arriving home had some of the shine knocked off it first thing next morning. In time-honoured fashion Mike brought me all the post to open (I open all letters in our household). Amongst the post-bag was a letter from a friend announcing that she was pregnant. As I read this, her news struck me as a hammer blow. I couldn't tell Mike, just pass him the letter to read for himself. He made no comment, leaving me to come to terms with it for myself.

Throughout our childlessness, some of the most difficult times have been watching contemporaries become pregnant and produce offspring. When I married, it was fun to attend the weddings of many friends, whilst learning, through various channels, of old school and college friends, with whom I had long since lost contact, being married. We all seemed to be in it together. Obviously, those same folk began to start families as we had planned to. Their success highlighted our own failure, the more so because of the close proximity of our ages and circumstances. I felt increasingly left behind and excluded from their experiences. Visiting school friends with their children, on occasions I have found myself at a loss to know what to say when the conversation has frequently concentrated on nappies, baby foods, sleepless nights, etc.

Interestingly, unlike some infertile women, I have never avoided the company of babies or children. In fact, I seek it out. Recently, a friend gave birth to her first child, and I learnt about it from mutual contacts. It became evident to me at least over the ensuing weeks that I was being carefully screened from contact with the new born child. Eventually, I approached the mum in question and asked if she was deliberately trying to be sensitive. She admitted that she was. I carefully explained that I did not begrudge her her child, but would feel leper-like if I was denied ready access to her or if the conversation were directed away from concentrating on her every time I entered the room. With these words, the situation naturally resolved itself. Though childless ourselves, we do not want to ruin the fun of being in the company of children of all ages. Indeed, every few years we seek to go on holiday with a family so that we can do the mad things you do with children. Summer 1987 saw us sunning ourselves in Ibiza together with Ishmael, Irene his wife, and Jos, Dan and Suzie, their three children. It was great fun and we appreciated the way that the youngsters accepted us and included us so readily. In fact, we see 'Ish', etc quite regularly, living so near them. One time when we were still the proud owners of a 2 CV6, we popped over, collected the boys and Ish and went to pick up a take-away meal. As we climbed into the car to return home, they noticed that the car was a soft-top and asked if the roof opened. When we said it did they requested a demonstration. We were convinced of their earnestness and, in spite of the fact that it was raining, we agreed, rolled back the roof and off we went. The boys stuck their heads out of the now open roof and had a great laugh— a major talking point for a number of days, according to Ish. Now we would never have done that for just the two of us. You need the company of children to ensure you do the mad things that make life worth living.

We have found it essential to build friendships with children in the families we have contact with. Maybe it keeps us young; it certainly keeps us in touch with how young people are thinking and enables Mike to prove himself a sporting superstar before an admiring audience. Mike's love for children is irrepressible, and I should never have forgiven myself had my sensitivities robbed him of the pleasure of playing with children, albeit the offspring of friends rather than our own.

Christmas loomed and I was not regaining my strength as quickly as I thought I would or as quickly as I wanted to. We organized an 'invitation' to my brother and sister-in-law's, where we would have the company of their two sons as well as my mother and father. Obviously I would be able to take it easy there and not offend anyone with my non-performance. Mike was anxious for me to choose a dress for Christmas and he escorted me on a shopping expedition. Normally I love trailing around shops—just looking and dreaming. This time it was all I could do to concentrate on the job in hand. He selected three dresses for me to try on. I made my choice and was keen to return home, even forgoing our customary cup of coffee, a part of every shopping ritual. Strangely, I found myself very self-conscious in the communal changing-room, convinced my stomach protruded unnaturally and fearful that someone would crash into my scar. For a number of weeks, I found myself very protective towards my stomach and fearful of doing harm to the wound, which was in fact well and truly sealed. The one long-term disappointment about my operation concerned my stomach. As a teenager, I had worked really hard at controlling my stomach muscles, so that I was proud of the flatness of my stomach. Ever since the operation, this control has been greatly impaired, much to my distress!

Christmas sped past—a great family time. We slept in the attic room at the top of my brother's house—a major effort to climb up to it and descend from it each day. The New Year saw us back in Leeds celebrating with friends and fellowship. I began to participate a lot more and grow less conscious of my perceived vulnerability.

DIARY

January 1ST 1983 New year, new baby! How often I had welcomed the arrival of the new year with these words. I've had the surgery; now I'll have the baby. I'm so looking forward to this year. Can't wait to tell Mike I'm pregnant. Mapping it all out in my mind. Hospital treatment wasn't so high a price to pay for our family, our twins.

To the Sales—purchased colour television with teletext. Great excitement, our first colour TV. Never spent so much money in one go, I don't think. Will think of Australia whenever I watch it. Sorry not to have made the trip. Still, grateful of the financial reserves so that we can get the tele. Convalescence much more acceptable with a colour Moron's Magnet to gaze at!

Mike will be home for much of the time, since he had booked holiday for Australia. Appreciate having him around so much. Quite strange in a way, not the normal experience of our married life to date.

Frustrated Mike won't let me do more. Forget

I'm not to lift. Caught me carting chairs across the room. He must be spying on me, springing out when I'm at a disadvantage.

January 1983 My first hospital appointment since operation. Mike accompanies me to Outpatients Department. Bit like a reunion meeting seeing all the women, or a good proportion of them, from my time on the ward. Amazing the sense of camaraderie we retain.

Appointment routine but will have to face the Pill question head-on. Don't want to go back on it—Mike supportive. Will the specialist insist? I'm not sure how much fight I have within me!

Left Mike in waiting-room, ascended stairs and entered the examination-room. Sighed with relief when the doctor pronounced all was well and that the wound was healing very well. Following this, question time began. Mr Hancock enquires after our sex life—cheeky, I thought! It was good to be able to tell him sex had resumed—a little cautiously at first; I'm not sure if Mike or I was the more diffident to start with.

Wasn't pressed hard over issue of Pill. Stood my ground and said I didn't want to go on the Pill. Drew upon every excuse I could think of: interfered with emotions, anxious about long-term effects on health, etc. Returned to Mike, relieved that I wasn't on the Pill and could concentrate on becoming pregnant. Made further appointment for July. I'd return then with a bulge, I felt sure.

COMMENTARY

The year after surgery was extremely odd. By March, I was physically very much better. Recovery had been slower than I had expected; activity tired me swiftly and it took a while to gain sufficient confidence not to walk with a stoop. However, it was not just my physique that was affected. The greatest and most enduring impact was upon my emotions. For no apparent reason, I'd burst into tears. I was particularly sensitive—maybe hypersensitive—and reacted strongly to comments people made, often quite unreasonably. The difficulty was that I was not aware that I was being particularly sensitive, so it proved difficult to do much about it. On one weekend of ministry Mike was unusually provocative during the evening ministry. Next morning, we ran into the criticisms over breakfast and it was all too much for me. Mike having given his all the evening before and aware that my calm exterior was masking an erupting volcano, excused us from breakfast, and back in our room the two of us exploded—I collapsed in tears; Mike lost his temper. Fortunately, others were handling the meetings that day; Mike would never have run them effectively.

It took about a year for my emotions to settle down again. Apparently, gynaecological operations do severely affect one's emotional condition. In reviewing my experiences, I do believe it would have helped us both to have been forewarned of the emotional traumas we could expect.

As time passed, life resumed its regular pattern: Mike travelling; myself taking responsibility for his secretarial work as necessary. During this time, I was quickly losing heart over the fact that I was not instantly pregnant. I had continued to utilize the Billings Method and was using the data on my temperature to determine when we should make love. This was OK until one day Mike let fly with an uncharacteristic outburst:

'I cannot make love to order!'

Aiming to have intercourse at the strategic time in my cycle had robbed our love-making of all its spontaneity. It was as though we were engaged in a military campaign, sex by numbers, 'Let's be 'aving you, lovely boy'; good successful procreation, conception confirmed. We decided to stop the temperature charts, etc and just have intercourse when we wanted. Once we did, I suddenly realized how tense I had become; focusing all my hopes and expectations on the evening dictated by my temperature. Mike also acknowledged how wound up he had become—hence the outburst. A new joy, excitement and pleasure came into our love-making. Foreplay was extensive and is as important as the act itself, this latter having dominated when conception was the foremost aim of sex.

Throughout our infertile years, we have become aware at different points of how intrusive to our relationship the treatment has become. Losing sight of each other, every nerve and sinew strains to perform in such a way that the long-awaited family will emerge. On each of these

occasions, we have had to step in directly and re-
assess where we are, who we are and what we are
looking for in our marriage. Children are always
only a part of marriage. My relationship with
Mike must always remain a higher priority over
that with my children—without that they would
not be effectively parented. Theory to date but
one to which we are committed. These times of
re-assessment were very important. We reassured
each other of our love and commitment. We were
forced into a position where we had to put our
childlessness into perspective. Hidden fears,
anxieties and tensions were freely expressed, and
once expressed, often evaporated. The greatest
lesson throughout was not to lose sight of love-
making for its own sake—giving pleasure to one
another. Enjoying the special physical privileges
marriage gives for their own sake. Inadvertently,
I had been rejecting Mike—'not tonight, darling,
my temperature is not right' (a unique excuse for
ladies world-wide!)—and he was also punishing
himself, feeling a failure every time he failed to
impregnate me. Strange are the many tributaries
we discover and wander down while flowing with
the mainstream of childlessness.

Easter brought our annual trip to Spring
Harvest. This was the most difficult time of year
for me, confronted by so many new babies and
new pregnancies. In fact, Spring Harvest to my
mind marks the year's beginning and end; our
diary revolves around it, and so I count off
another twelve months of disappointment: still no
baby for me.

Returning from Spring Harvest, I entered what was to prove the lowest state I have ever reached. It was about five months since my operation and still nothing had stirred, not even a miscarriage. For the first time, I felt as if nothing ever would and if it wouldn't, life could go take a running jump at itself. If I couldn't have my babies, I certainly wasn't interested in living. What cause had I for laughter, joy, friendship? Everything within me wanted to swing a heavy door shut on existence, bolt it solidly and stay shut up doing nothing. I became obsessed with my ovulation thermometer once again. I could see the stress written across Mike's face. He began to work ever harder but with little heart.

June arrived with all the scent and promise of summer. However, I for one was not warmed. A deep depression settled upon me. It was as though I was buried, literally buried under tons of rubble. I felt enclosed; my mind was both obsessed with children and crushed, as though caught in a vice. I had never experienced depression before, it was hateful; I was hateful; what was I to do?

Each morning I could think of no good reason to get up. Poorly motivated, I only got out of bed and dressed because of Mike's insistence. I also lost contact with Mike—we didn't fall out, it was just that even his humour, care, anger didn't touch me. It seemed distant in a way and irrelevant to my situation. Love-making, the only sure way to secure a pregnancy, ceased altogether.

I could not talk about childlessness and grew

both over-sensitive and intolerant towards other people. I avoided contact with them on the subject as well. My relationship with God was left to continue as best it could. One occasion, I let fly a tirade in his direction, which I realize he patiently endured and washed away my tears with his own.

Mid-July, following Mike's prompting, I phoned a friend who had suffered infertility before recently conceiving and producing a child of her own. Throughout the phone call, all I could hear were the happy sounds of her child playing in the background. Not especially welcome. After I had poured out my heart, she sought to comfort me and encourage me, praying with me before ending the call. I replaced the receiver and howled and howled, long and hard. I was not through this bleak period but just expressing myself honestly to someone I knew appreciated the pain of infertility did help. Beneath it all, I recognised I had to come through the pain barrier. This was my fight—it was to prove a wearisome conflict.

Slowly, over a three-month period, all the accumulated pain, anger, bitterness, frustration and hurt rose up and confronted me. As I wrestled within the depths of depression, the sole same question constantly flashed before me. Would I accept, come to terms with my current childlessness or not? Just because I couldn't conceive, life went on regardless and I could either join in, limping if necessary, or bury my head in my hands and allow it to pass me by. Such a position was I knew untenable since it would be the height of selfishness. But it was not an easy decision to come to, nor one I was convinced I would make in the midst of the trauma.

Mike is fond of quoting from speeches of famous individuals—one such that sticks in my mind is from a speech of John F. Kennedy. It runs, 'When written in Chinese, the word "crisis" is composed of two characters. One represents danger and the other represents opportunity.' This was my situation. My crisis would either be a situation which could well destroy me, and maybe my husband and marriage with me, or it could present an opportunity for developing character and discovering how to live with disadvantage.

It provided a potent illustration of powerlessness. Try as I might, there was no way I could alter my circumstances. I was powerless and dependent upon forces external to myself. We in the West are rarely placed in such a situation—unlike so many who share a common humanity world-wide. Since that dark hour, this thought of powerlessness has provoked us to think far more extensively about the quality of life of so many and to look at God's will for them. His heart is overflowing with love and compassion, and he looks to the church to express this.

Throughout these bleak months, the arrival of my period took me to the lowest depths. Realizing that I was not pregnant once again was devastating. I never seemed prepared for the realization. I would cry and feel desperately miserable, feelings which were encouraged by the hormonal state of my body at that time.

Mike was at his wits' end. He worked away in his own inimitable fashion, covered hundreds of miles and steered me through the crisis as best he could. All decision making fell to him and certainly the ordering of the house was woefully neglected, so absorbed was I with myself. I would not have guessed at the degree of Mike's frustration, he never being one to rock what he perceives to be an already unstable boat. Only as I recovered and returned to the land of the living did I discover the despair he had experienced. Throughout we realized on reflection that we had proved Scripture: 'Love bears all things, believes all things, hopes all things, endures all things. Love never ends' (1 Cor 13:7-8, Revised Standard Version). Ours had and it hasn't!

Chapter Eight

July saw me back at the Outpatients Department. I was shocked to be seen by an unknown doctor, unknown to me at least. He seemed ignorant of my history and asked very basic questions. He concluded what I knew already: my physical condition was fine. However, no question was asked or comment made about my emotional state. If the truth were known, I was in pieces and that afternoon the pieces multiplied.

I left the examination-room with the words 'keep trying and relax!' ringing in my ears. Relax! Farcical—the harder I tried, the more wound up I became. Relaxing is not something you can simply turn on by the flick of some psychological switch. It's rather like telling a manic-depressive to pull himself together. The advice may have grains of truth wrapped up in it but it's a foreign language as far as providing any help is concerned. Why hadn't I seen a doctor who was aware of my case? Someone might have read the notes at least! As I departed, a further appointment was made for April 1984.

Even as I emerged from my position of despair, I remained emotionally unstable, tearful at the drop of a hat. Friends were so very understanding and supportive over this period. I am so grateful Jesus left us not only his word and his Spirit but also each other! It was difficult to say what might provoke me to cry: tears of grief or tears of rage or just simply tears. All I can say is these outbursts were upon me all of a sudden and I simply expressed myself in sobs. I don't believe there would be much benefit from close analysis—but I'm grateful I was accepted for who and what I was over these months. Mike was always supportive; to my relief, showed no signs of public embarrassment; never criticized or pressurized me to be other than who I was. Unfortunately, he continued to refuse to allow my tears to deteriorate into bouts of self-pity, identifying these with an annoying consistency.

Christmas 1983 saw us with Mike's family. There were no young children around, which was helpful at this stage. As I recovered possession of my emotions, I remained somewhat vulnerable and the atmosphere of Christmas with excited youngsters and dewy-eyed parents would have proved too much, perhaps. It is amazing how aware one becomes of the association of festivals with children. Mike and I have spent Christmas on our own—I'm sure it was never designed to be spent in that way!

Having said as much, it reminds us of all those who do have to spend Christmas alone: the number I have no knowledge of, but it is probably large. We are becoming used to the phrase 'disadvantaged people.' This can apply to the physically disabled, the mentally ill, the unemployed, the West Indian and Asian communities, the urban poor—broadly, anyone with a disadvantage! It is also taught clearly that God's heart is full of compassion for those who suffer—physically, emotionally, mentally or spiritually—and the church as God's expression on earth should reflect that compassion.

However, it is also evident that the disadvantaged are generally noticeable by their absence from our congregations—that is those we would immediately recognize as disadvantaged. This is an issue to which the church needs to pay urgent attention but is not the subject of this book. And yet, within congregations up and down the country, there are those who are disadvantaged, feel themselves to be so, and yet who are not offered the fellowship and friendship that could meet them realistically in their place of pain, confusion, self-deprecation, etc. We have, for example, the single parent, the child with only a father or a mother, the divorced, the elderly, etc, etc.

We need to ask ourselves: 'Do we have a theology for all these areas of disadvantage?' Further: 'Do we act after the character and fashion of Jesus in response to such folk?' We have little to say to a fragmenting society if we speak from a homogeneous platform; ours is a visual age. Church life can provide, should provide, the visual confirmation of our numerous verbal messages.

As a childless couple, we at times feel disadvantaged. Disadvantaged in the sense of isolated from the pack; non-contributory in the expected way. Where were our kids? As we travel to different places it is assumed we have children. 'How are the children?' Or 'How many children do you have?' These are frequently posed questions. On replying we have none, the most common reply is, 'Oh! You don't have any children?' I refrain from verbalizing my inner thoughts at such a moment: 'That is a most accurate summary of what I've just said'; 'What devastating intellect!'

The attitude, however, runs from confusion to a hint of criticism. I believe in the days of yuppies the criticism is the assumption that we have chosen to be a career couple and hence deliberately chosen not to have children. How often we live in the conviction of our assumptions rather than truth. It is wearisome to recount the fact that we are childless. And yet sometimes in the face of tonal criticism, one feels obliged to launch into a defensive justification. It is difficult not to—the sense of being misunderstood and apparently judged is almost too great a burden to bear on top of the ever-present desire for children.

As we age, gracefully I trust, we find ourselves in a strange no man's land. Old enough and married long enough for us to have reproduced in the normal course of affairs, we see our peer group wrapped up in playing mummies and daddies, which we quite obviously are not. This re-focuses their point of interest and naturally draws them together with other parents—often further friends who find themselves equally occupied with offspring.

'Well you have your independence—no dependants!' folk announce. Yes, we do. However, mixing with those some considerable number of years younger than ourselves, their passion for pubs, parties and peripatetic lifestyle—the calling and culture of youth—leaves us somewhat frustrated and unfulfilled. We are in the age bracket of the dinner-party and passionate-debate set. Our flexibility created through our infertility is of great advantage in many ways—but only in as far as we first come to terms with our childlessness! Nothing is advantageous until you can first see the nature of the advantage. So often we are quick to identify a neighbour or friend's advantage, while sadly complaining about our lot. Such is the paradox of our human condition.

We have talked with a good number of childless couples who feel adrift in an uncharted sea when it comes to church life. Some find it very difficult to inform others of their childlessness. It appears that there is something of an evangelical stigma against those who cannot 'go forth and multiply'. It's as though four children (the standard evangelical number) were *de rigueur* in fulfilling one's commitment to God and his call to world mission. Sometimes the very expression 'we are childless' in response to a question about children completely embarrasses the enquirer. The subject is changed or there is an awkward silence, maybe punctuated by a non-comprehending 'I see'! I well remember talking with those who found themselves unemployed in the early days of the present malaise. They expressed a sense of feeling like outcasts from society. For example, if at a party the conversation turned, as it naturally does, to the nature of work individuals were engaged in, when they expressed they were unemployed, it produced a pointed full stop to the conversation. People felt uncomfortable, unsure of where to turn in conversational terms in the face of such a statement. We were untrained, badly socialized when it came to responding to the unemployed, even in the realm of words. And so it is so often with the childless.

I can appreciate the difficulties—how should someone react to my childlessness? With pity? With sorrow? With humour? With an anecdote? I've met them all. I would suggest that no one should react to my childlessness but continue to react and respond to me! A statement such as 'I've not met someone who can't have children before', or 'That must prove very tough. How do *you* handle it?' is quite satisfactory and gives me an opportunity to continue in conversation without any sense of embarrassment. My co-conversationalist has established a bridge for me to walk across.

Childless couples need to be included in

activities. If they can cope with children around them, then invite them to participate in family life. Unfortunately, in these days of nuclear families the lives are far more intense. In an extended family one can retreat from the immediate proximity of the youngsters to chat with the elder statesman. It is an easier framework. Hence the church provides an ideal forum for the childless, as for all disadvantaged people, or it should do. As a church, we must develop this area. Concentrate on socializing as much as worshipping or preaching.

It may well prove constructive to put childless couples in touch with each other. Forming a basic self-help group can be very constructive. At times it may generate a sense of desperation and powerlessness—most self-help groups do at times lock into the negatives, relating to their particular circumstances—but it will also widen couples' horizons through walking in the shoes of others in their predicament as well as provide a forum for generating ideas, from handling the medical aspects to socializing enjoyably. Such a group must never become isolated from the main body of the fellowship—it is only ever one of the numerous groups meeting which together add up to the church locally.

Perhaps the hardest thing of all is to hear those mothers (and to a lesser extent, fathers) who continually complain about children. It is self-evident that caring for children is time consuming and energy sapping. There are obvious frustrations inherent with parenthood, as with every circumstance life draws us into. However, to be told that one is better off without kids when to conceive and give birth is one's deepest desire is not a constructive comment. It may well involve something of a truism—but one might just as well tell an unemployed individual how fortunate he is not to have the stress of management to contend with. Every situation produces its own unique pressures. My pain may appear to be a blessing from your perspective. But then that is only your perspective. Our task is to express commitment to one another by discovering points of contact which themselves generate love, acceptance and support. Let's get to it and prove in some measure the competence of the gospel in the life of God's church.

Having completed our customary eighteen months in one location, we were on the move again. Mike, having joined the leadership team of BYFC, was finding communications difficult with all the rest based in the south. So we set forth from Leeds and settled in Banstead—in a lovely rented flat, part of a large house set in beautiful grounds. The stillness and quiet was such that for several nights, we found it hard to fall asleep, used to the background noise of buses, lorries changing gear and revellers singing as they staggered home from the working men's club situated a few doors away from our Leeds residence.

Of course, moving required that we move our medical records. However, I felt I must be on the verge of conceiving, so neglected to make the necessary arrangements. With great assurance, I cancelled my April appointment at the Leeds General Infirmary and cut us free from hospitals —or so I thought!

We moved in the February and were hardly settled before undertaking the annual pilgrimage to Spring Harvest. That year we ran a seminar entitled, 'How to Pray with your Partner'. We were amazed at how popular this proved. As part of our presentation, we mentioned our childlessness and our relationship with God in the midst of such pain. I found it difficult going public—and at that stage had to leave Mike to do the talking: I should have cried had I tried! However, just mentioning our situation drew a number of childless couples around us and it was a joy to be able to talk and pray with them. All were at different points along the journey we had made; some had reached their wonderful destination. They had children following years of pain, disappointment and even despair.

Twenty-nine-years-old—and childless. I'd always promised myself kids by the time I was thirty! It was a very large mountain to climb. Strange how our own preconditions can become cruel rods beating upon our backs. I felt distinctly miserable. What was I to do?

Mike travelled to Nigeria with BYFC in February 1985. On my own with time to think, I determined to take up a challenge. Entirely on my own initiative, I enrolled in a secretarial training course at Pitman's, Wimbledon. Three months intensive training would see me able to run offices, take down shorthand, word process and type exceptionally quickly. I felt a distinct 'buzz' from the thought of such a course. I wondered what Mike would say.

I also took a trip to the doctor's and requested taking up my treatment for infertility where I'd left off. A brief account of my gynaecological history so far and he immediately recommended me to a London hospital: the Hammersmith, famed for the exploits of Mr Robert Winston and his pioneering work in In Vitro Fertilization. I felt something of a VIP as I left the surgery. I was going to consult The Mr Robert Winston. Strange what ridiculous things enhance our feelings of self-worth, or is it just self-importance?

Poor Mike! As he arrived at Heathrow following a most traumatic departure from Kano, Nigeria, I immediately off-loaded all my news as we travelled back to Banstead in the car. For years, Mike has gently (and not so gently) tried to educate me in holding back my news until he is unwound and relaxed. So often as he has returned home from work, I have found myself pouring out my heart on half-a-dozen issues I've faced even before he has got his coat off. His response? Tetchy, sulky and angry. But I find it difficult not to talk about those things of the most immediate consequence to me the moment we are together. The joys of marriage!

Fortunately, we were not alone on this car journey. As I informed Mike excitedly about my enrolment at secretarial college and of further infertility treatment, all he could do was mouth platitudinous statements: 'How nice', 'That's good'. Hardly the reasoned, wise counsel of a man of God. I do believe he was shell-shocked by my barrage of news and left stunned. Only when we arrived home and were on our own did I realize that he was in desperate need of emotional nourishment, and unable to respond rationally to anything until I had met him at his point of need. With this realization, I felt a bit of a heel; but also a bit deflated because there had been so poor a response to my obvious excitement.

Over the next few days, I got the response I needed. Mike was thrilled at the secretarial course. More because I had gone out on my own and initiated something. Also I suspect because the government were paying, courtesy of the TOPS scheme. With regard to the infertility treatment, he was supportive but not enthusiastic. It was not until sometime later he confessed why. He feared this would place an intolerable burden of unhappiness upon me. He had observed the emotional traumas of earlier treatments and, accurately as it happens, foresaw the clouds of desperation gathering ready to surround me, us, once this further treatment got under way. His support was all I needed. We pursued further treatment.

A month passed, no contact from the Hammersmith. I phoned the doctor—'These things take time,' he responded, but referred me to Kings College Hospital as well. They offered an appointment there for the beginning of May.

Spring Harvest came and went again. Remembered notably for two low points. One friend announced her pregnancy; the other that she had been accepted for a test-tube baby. My emotions ran riot: downhill in a disorderly direction!

Returning home, I began my secretarial course. Something of a fillip. Discovering I was the second oldest in my class was only borne by comforting myself that I was not the oldest. The majority were school and college leavers—none had children. The atmosphere was refreshing and fun. Full of vitality and energy. Having been a teacher, I enjoyed being the other side of the desk again; and emerged with a comprehensive understanding of the Friday-afternoon syndrome.

Another feature of my undertaking this secretarial course was that it introduced Mike and me to role reversal. He tailored his diary so that he was working from home and not away. Waving me farewell each morning, he would vacuum, clean, shop and cook. He did this well; rather too well. My insecurities came to the fore. I didn't like this stranger organizing my kitchen, cooking all the meals, budgeting the housekeeping. We entertain frequently and I would arrive home to find the flat filled with wonderful aromas. When guests arrived, Mike seated us all at the table and slipped in and out of the kitchen, producing mouth-watering dish after mouth-watering dish! I was alarmed. Was I now redundant? Strange feelings of insecurity swept over me as I watched Mike perform what had been my role traditionally.

Worst of all, he was really enjoying himself. I must confess the household expenditure rose considerably. Mike maintained, with a wicked grin on his face, that running a home only entailed two hours' work a day. Why did I, and others, make so much fuss? I contented myself and abused him by pointing out the fact that he did no ironing; a point he readily admitted and continues to resist correcting.

My appointment at Kings entailed taking an afternoon off from my course. Mike collected me in the car and we undertook the tiresome drive across London's southern sector to Denmark Hill.

The Gynaecology and Endocrinology Unit was on the fifth floor of a modern block right alongside the maternity unit! As we sat, with others, waiting to see our specialist, we gazed with unbelieving eyes upon an area where pregnant women joyfully waddled, waiting for the first signs of the onset of labour. Looking away to the walls, one was confronted by photographs picturing 'miracle' babies whose stories were contained in letters pinned next to them, all from couples who had at some stage sat where we were now.

Eventually, we were summoned to meet our new doctor. He was the endometriosis specialist. The nature of my treatment at Leeds had obviously directed us into his province. His belief was that my endometriosis had regenerated itself —recommended next step laparoscopy number two. The earliest mutually convenient date proved to be September and I booked in. It was suggested to Mike that he do further sperm counts—he declined.

We left, picked up a leaflet on 'the morning after pill', took the lift to the entrance hall and were glad to step through the doors into the warmth of the sun. As we walked towards the car, an air of gloom descended. Neither of us talked for quite some time. Each knew what the other was feeling. A sense of despondency. Had we the energy to engage in another bout of treatment? Just being in the atmosphere of the infertility unit had heightened the sense of grief at being childless. Even the sun failed to cheer our sinking spirits. It was as though a wound which had apparently knit together had opened up again. We were sore; raw. And neither of us had the capacity to meet the other's need.

It is amazing that at times such as those the saddest refrains run repeatedly through the mind. I felt isolated yet again; crushed by circumstances beyond my immediate control. Tears were in my eyes, as I knew they would be in Mike's too, and yet both of us lacked the energy to cry; what difference could our tears make?

Eventually, as we talked, we realized that the path we were now treading could eventually give us the children we so keenly desired. At the same time it could prove to be a disappointing cul-de-sac.

This time we knew the score. We knew what emotional resources would be called upon. We were entering with our eyes open. As for me, although I felt burdened with sadness, I did not feel the weight of depression settling upon me. I had little appetite for further hospitalization and treatment and yet I could yield to it while retaining a rational, even detached perspective. This was new. As we walked, I quietly committed my path into the hand of God—this time he squeezed my hand—and I knew deep within he was here with me. While I remained saddened and disturbed outwardly, a rich peacefulness, a tranquility, a sense of stillness surrounded the very core of my being; the essential me. I could proceed.

Mike wanted to cease the treatment at this stage. He tried to talk me out of going on. However, my mind was made up. In fact, Mike was quite agitated; hurting over our childlessness; also hurting over the fact that I would have to face more investigations. I came to recognise how dear to him I was—how distraught he felt at apparently abandoning me to the surgeon's knife and all that would entail.

I was touched by his anguish. Whichever way he turned, he faced anguish: that of childlessness on the one hand, my physical pain on the other. A no-win situation. One where he had to find for himself the reality of God. Something he did and for which I was most grateful.

This period of treatment was to prove the most distressing and also the last. It also marked that point on our voyage where we discovered that we were whole individuals, in spite of our infertility; that we were complete as a couple, even without children of our own; that God loved us, had called us and was everything to us, although our con-

stant *cri de coeur* was as yet apparently unheeded.
We needed this final chapter.

Chapter Nine

Hospital again! Not my favourite place. And I knew Mike's preference for my not attending had been heightened through the fiasco of checking in, as described earlier. Normally, I steel myself sufficiently well to cope with most circumstances. This was something else altogether.

We had recently moved yet again! This time to Chichester, where we intend to stay for some time. Obviously, the hospital in London was some miles away from our home and we were grateful to Jonathan and Sarah Markham for providing us with a short-stay home within easy reach of the hospital.

Fairly emotional from having just moved home, I could not believe the situation I encountered on the ward. Having been unable to book in immediately, once in my bed, I discovered that the bedside radio wasn't working. In fact it hadn't worked for quite some time, the same as other people's on the same ward. For all who appreciate the pleasure a radio brings when there are long hours to kill, this proved a major blow. However, this was just the start!

I soon learnt that the TV was broken, so all ward entertainment was left to the individual. Bored and frustrated, I determined to phone Mike. Well, you guessed it. A nurse apologetically informed me that the phone was not functioning. I had neither the energy nor the confidence to wander the hospital clad in no more than my nightdress in search of an operational Payphone. Miserable and angry, I set my sights on visiting time. I should then get Mike to take up my case—after all, his role at the Evangelical Alliance involved campaigns on occasions.

When Mike arrived to visit, I was delighted to see him. He could not believe my tale of woe, which had been added to by having to attempt consuming a poor curry, the order for which I had the previous occupant in my bed to thank. I could see he wanted to make some form of complaint but did not know where to turn. The nurses, the front-line troops and hence in the immediate firing line, had been absolutely super and most apologetic at the current state of affairs. It seemed unrealistic to let fly at them and to his credit Mike refrained.

We prayed for the day to come which would see me in the operating theatre, always supposing it was operational! before Mike left for what I learnt was a very restless night. Thinking that my day of troubles was at an end, I was rudely returned to reality when requested to leave my bed, gather my personal belongings and make my way to the men's ward. The reason? So that the female ward could be closed for the night and hence would not need to be staffed. As I made my way into the men's ward, I thought, I'm not sure this is the sort of thing mother approves of! Next morning, of course, the whole procedure was reversed and I returned to the female ward.

The laparoscopy went ahead as planned. Mike had insisted that I be released from the hospital that same evening, not willing that I should stay an hour longer than necessary. We were so grateful for a temporary home so close, in that the hospital could not object on mileage grounds. However, we had to wait until the doctor had seen us and given us news of the op. and officially released me from his charge. Visiting time passed and Mike doggedly stayed on. Other patients had to change wards and eventually so did we, my clothes and personal effects remaining behind and locked in the now empty female ward.

Eventually, at 9.30 p.m. the tired doctor appeared in the doorway of the ward. I was relieved, having begun to feel just a little awkward at standing out for going home that evening. At that point I relaxed; too soon.

The news was good. The endometriosis had not regenerated; a victory for prayer and faith, if somewhat disappointing for the endometriosis specialist who was giving us this news. Now it seemed the problem was adhesions across the entrance to the tubes which prevented them from collecting eggs during ovulation. These adhesions were in fact the result of my earlier tubal surgery. 'Spit the dog,' I thought, or words to that effect. The wave of relief in knowing that the endo-metriosis was not in my system any longer broke on the rocks of despair with this news that I still couldn't fall pregnant.

More surgery was a possibility. This would again be major laser surgery to split the ad-hesions. The doctor informed me that he had split as many adhesions as he could during my time in theatre. As Mike and I were reeling with this information, the doctor casually added:

'I can offer you a test-tube baby if you like.'

We mumbled something in response, our hearts set on just getting out of the hospital to somewhere more conducive to reflection and calm conversation. I dressed and allowed Mike to deftly steer me out of the hospital, into the car and back to the welcome home of Jonathan and Sarah. They were themselves a childless couple, so there was an immediate affinity between us. It was good to be off the ward and in a comfortable bed with Mike by my side. Even if he did look stupid trying to sleep motionless for fear of hit-ting my wound!

We now had to face the whole issue of In Vitro Fertilization; test-tube babies. What were our thoughts on this subject, so current in the news? Had we got clear ideas or just faint options in the light of all that we had absorbed?

In fact, we had done some thinking around this

subject. This had not been technical but rather in the light of our Christian faith and our own personal feelings. It has always been our view that human life begins from conception and we have great problems with abortion. How one can pick an arbitrary point in a baby's development and claim that that is when life begins defeats me. Certainly Scripture supports the view that our humanity, the image of God that we bear, begins at the moment of conception. Hence, we hold to the position that the moment the egg is fertilized by the sperm, we are talking of a human being, who should enjoy all the rights afforded to a person in a civilized society.

As far as test-tube children were concerned, we had two major difficulties. Obviously, in any such treatment, it would involve my egg and Mike's sperm. We certainly would resist any treatment that sought to bring a third party into the arrangement, however anonymous their involvement might be. However, even though just Mike and I would be involved, we both wanted to know what would happen to those eggs that were fertilized and not implanted.

As it was explained to us, I would have around eight eggs removed from my ovary and these would be fertilized outside the womb before the four healthiest were implanted. No more than four would be implanted for fear of multiple births. So what of the four not implanted? These may have failed to grow, have developed unsatisfactorily or just been overlooked in the final choice. If these were then allowed to die, what does that say when one believes humanity begins from the moment of conception? Also as medical science progresses, we will reach a stage where it will be possible to keep such fertilized eggs alive for more extensive periods of time than at present. Will they then become the test ground for medical exploration? It seems that medical ethics is such a grey area, with very few clear reference points, that we are guaranteed very little in terms of personal involvement in the future of fertilized eggs. This whole area is one that requires far more open debate, involving theologians and philosophers as well as medics. It seems strange that such vital ethical and philosophical issues are left to the medical profession to solve on their own!

Our second major concern was the amount of money being invested in both research into this field of medicine and into the performance of the necessary courses of treatment. Painful though it might be, the facts are that childlessness is not a disease. It is a part of life. A society that suggests, as ours does, that the blight of infertility must be removed at all costs is one that could be accused of having taken leave of its senses. When cancer, kidney disease, etc, etc runs riot, we are prepared to pour millions of pounds into providing wish fulfilment. One might, with some justification, ask why such large sums of money are not being made available to the legion of unemployed in our country to enable them to fulfil their wishes. I must confess to a high degree of suspicion over such vast expenditure in this area and wonder what the real fascination with the technology of life creation stems from.

Both Mike and I are tired of constantly watching interviews on the television with couples who maintain that to be childless is the worst blight to fall on anybody's household. All I can imagine is that they either go through life blinkered or that they are exceptionally selfish, with their life ordered entirely around their wants. Why are there no interviews with couples such as ourselves who have an altogether different perspective, equally valid? It almost appears that the media wants to endorse a particular point of view which is always bad news for any society that would like to pride itself on its freedoms, especially freedom of speech. But that's another book altogether!

IVF is not as wonderful as it sounds. Only 8.9% of treatment episodes (cycles) conclude with a couple having a live baby, according to the voluntary listening authority's 1986 figures. This is an average figure across twenty-five clinics. Such clinics can have waiting lists of two to three years. Be aware of the potential disappointments.

With such views we feel that we could not proceed with a test-tube baby for ourselves and have appreciated all that we have discovered in continuing childless. We have discovered that character is built into our individual lives and into the nature of our marriage through facing this one issue honestly. We can only speak of the kindness and goodness of God throughout. A situation which had the capacity to control and shape us has rather proved a touchstone in our own development, and we know that we are the richer as a result. We can concentrate on investing that richness back into the world of which we are a part and into the lives of people who cross our path. As you have read our testament of childlessness, I trust that you have emerged the richer.

Appendix

Katey and I decided not to adopt. For us that is the right decision. However, for many, adoption proves a happy path to fulfilling parental ambitions, and we are so grateful to our friends Jonathan and Sarah Markham for providing their personal story as an appendix to this book.

God provides for all our needs—emotional, spiritual, physical and psychological—in many diverse ways. For Jonathan and Sarah adoption was his divine option.

★ ★ ★

'That's the way I shall have to have children if I get married.' With these words I discovered that my girlfriend, upon whom I already had designs, was unable to bear children. At the age of sixteen, Sarah was informed that since she had not developed ovaries she would not suffer the discomfort of monthly periods, but neither would she be able to carry a child of her own. To me this was one of the most devastating blows of my life. Everyone who knew me was unable to avoid my overwhelming love of children, and it was immediately obvious how much I longed to have my own. Initially I looked at her as if there was something wrong with her and felt both sorry for her and angry with God. Why had he arranged this for me?

We had heard that you had to demonstrate three years of stable marriage before you were considered for adoption and that the wait from acceptance to the placing of a child was also about three years. Logic suggested that since we did not need to go through the process of demonstrating medically our infertility, why not allow both three year periods to run concurrently? However, when we wrote with this suggestion to one of the only specifically Christian adoption agencies they were quick to inform us that this was not possible. To be told this in a pro forma letter (the first of many) was a great disappointment since we felt we had a good chance. We knew that at twenty-eight and twenty-six, age was not on our side (Jonathan particularly wanted to have children early) and so their unwillingness seemingly to consider what we saw as our unique circumstances was a blow.

However, God arranged a change of job for Jonathan involving a move of home up to London, and a new and very traumatic teaching job for Sarah which enabled three years to pass very quickly!

On our third wedding anniversary, once again a letter was penned to the afore-mentioned society with high hopes. The pro forma letter informing us that lists were closed was another blow. We then knew that there was nothing for it but to embark upon what we knew could be a very long letter-writing campaign. Booklets were obtained, a letter written, typed and duplicated (we could do the pro forma bit too!!) and despatched to every address we could find that might just consider us for a child. At this stage many well-meaning people told us just how much pressure local authorities and adoption agencies were under, and that some lists were only opened for one day a year. Only those whose letters arrived on that day got lucky. Somehow, however, we were not put off, telling each other that since we felt God had marked all this out for us he must have a way.

Pro formas galore plopped through the letter box saying, 'Sorry no babies,' 'Sorry lists closed,' or 'Sorry we can't help.' However, there was a ray of hope as one society asked if we would come and talk further and a local authority invited us to an information evening for prospective adopters. The contrast could hardly have been greater.

The adoption society interview consisted of three hours of intense personal conversation in which we began to explain our situation and feelings, and the social worker carefully explained the adoption process as they operated it. It is difficult to explain the value to us of that conversation, which although offering no false hopes, did not dismiss out of hand our longing for a new baby. We left, reeling with information, but encouraged that there could be light at the end of the tunnel. We now had to wait to hear if, on the strength of that conversation, the society was prepared to allow us to complete forms and begin the process of approval.

A few days later, and with somewhat higher expectations, we joined several couples like ourselves for an evening of information and discussion for prospective adopters. There we were told that if we were interested in babies they really weren't interested in us. Trendy social workers took time and technology to sell us children with special needs—teenagers with the desire to dismantle entire plumbing systems and youngsters with severe behavioural difficulties. The commitment and dedication of these folk to the children in their care and their potential was very moving, and many questions flooded into our minds, accompanied by a combination of sympathy and guilt along with a sense of uncertainty and inadequacy. Was this really what we should do? Were we selfish to want a healthy baby while so many were in need? We were Christians, after all, who were called to serve the needy. But we really wanted a little baby. Could we cope with a disabled child?

We left, feeling dejected and confused; filled with feelings and questions we did not know what to do with. However, then as always, there gradually returned the conviction that if God intended us to have a child he was going to work this out. After all, the first society had offered hope. We hung on to that hope through many more brown envelopes containing badly duplicated versions of the same bad news. Another local authority invited us to visit, and in a building decorated like a shop, with the photographs of needy children all over the walls, once again we were told that if we wanted a baby we were wasting our time. Had they forgotten us, we began to think?

At last, the joy of opening an envelope saying that the society panel had agreed to *begin* the process. So, in December 1983, 'the forms' came through the door and the work really began. Pages and pages of detailed searching questions requiring hours of thought. Yes, of course we had been asked on many forms before what we watched on television and whether we played any sport. But what was our attitude to money? What sort of family life would we provide for the child? How much did we know about child development, and how did we deal with disagreements with one another? Why should we have to satisfy someone else that we had the right answers? What answers were the right ones, and if they thought we had got them wrong would they refuse us a child?

Suddenly the big 'they' became a factor as we prepared to have our life, present and past, dissected, our home examined and our relationship and emotions put under the microscope. The selection of referees was made, and they were asked to write and be interviewed personally. This

long form and its contents rattle cages of uncertainty and insecurity and even at times infuri-
ation at what seemed an imposition. But we
longed for a baby and if this was the way . . . well.

Probably the most difficult questions related to
the child itself—many questions we had never
conceived of. What did we know about heredity,
let alone think about it? Were we prepared to take
a child from a different ethnic background, or
with physical or mental handicaps? But more important for us was a question which lay behind
them all: What right had we to make a choice of
this sort? Wasn't every child God's gift? Wouldn't
choosing be almost degrading?

The question of handicap raised doubts about
whether we could cope if something serious
happened to our child, if we were not prepared to
accept a disabled little one. These questions, along
with that of skin colour, raised questions and
differences between us; Jonathan being ready for
anything and Sarah being more cautious and
sensible. To know God's answer and to be at peace
with it was so important for us. Although our
married life, like most, had seen its ups and
downs, joys and tensions, the approach process
and results of adoption were characterized by an
almost unreal and improbable peace that can only
be described as miraculous. A simple trust and
degree of faith neither of us had found easy in
any other part of our lives was given to us at every
stage, and it was this that accompanied the docu-
menting of our decision not to accept a child with
a disability, as we were uncertain we could cope

with that choice, although we knew that should we have a child and he became ill or had an accident God would equip as necessary. Neither did we feel it right to accept a coloured child into our predominantly white lifestyle. Most of all, we wanted a little white healthy baby and although we expressed this, we also said we wished to remain as open as possible.

The envelope was sealed and despatched, and the examinations and interviews known as the home study began. At the time we were about to have the inside of our house rearranged, and we were most apprehensive about what the social worker would think. Hoping she would not decide that she could not place a child in a temporary building site, we nervously opened our door for the first of many visits. Far from the detailed survey we feared, a casual and interested glance in each room seemed to satisfy her that our little house was suitable to accommodate a child.

Then, more questions, but now they began to go both ways as we started to explore the background to what we hoped to do. Never had we realised that we had a 'history'. We knew something about our mother and father's childhood and about their parents, all things our baby would need to be told and to understand. We knew that the parents who brought us into the world loved us, but adopted children might struggle with that if their origins were difficult, for example, involving incest or where one or both parents had been in prison. The prospect of facing these and other issues like them filled us with the fear of giving wrong answers.

During this time we were constantly encouraged to get in touch with other adoptive parents, and we attended conferences arranged by the society and meetings of a parent organization. Our experience here was unusual as we found that the underlying peace and unexplainable certainty we felt about it all, left us strangely separate from the others, who seemed to have endless problems with their societies' social workers or other spheres of bureaucracy. Knowing that God would provide seemed to leave us somewhat insulated. We talked together of how we would like to share our peace and confidence with those of whom we met, but whenever the subject came up, our explanatiuons were greeted with the nods and smiles of total misunderstanding and we have not pursued our links with these groups.

Our church, along with our families, provided boundless interest, support and above all prayer as we went through the process. Eventually the visits were over, the referees' report complete and the medical examination satisfactory, and we awaited the final decision. Jonathan was away at a leadership conference with the Evangelical Alliance and Sarah was at home looking after two children when the letter arrived to say we were accepted and on the official list. This was eighteen months after the first letter began the process! The sense of relief and excitement was tremendous, but it soon ebbed away as we realized that the wait was still likely to be about two years. However, having realized that it would not help us to scrutinize the post and jump at every phone call, our lives continued. Twelve months, even fourteen and fifteen, passed quickly, but then the waiting began to get a little tedious and occasionally frustrated conversations occurred between us as to whether it would even happen.

Spring Harvest has become a major event in the lives of many of us, and Jonathan's involvement in exhibition organization meant he needed to be there for not only the three weeks of the event, but the week before and after. Many times we had joked about a little one arriving at this time. Jonathan had spent four days in Prestatyn, and rushed back to have two days at home, before embarking with a van for Minehead. One Monday evening, we sat down for supper with two close friends. The phone rang and Jonathan answered it. 'There's this little baby boy,' was about all that was remembered from a call that left supper cold on the table and three other people open-mouthed around it. This was the first we heard about the tiny three-week-old boy who before long was to change our lives.

A multitude of frantic phone calls to friends and family revealed another answer to a family prayer. Jonathan has two younger sisters both married. The older, Barbara, and her husband Jonnie had already given birth to two beautiful boys and another was on the way. Coming to terms with not producing the first grandchild, despite being the oldest and married first, had been difficult to swallow, but how we loved being with those boys. Judith, unbeknown to us, had been told she too was expecting despite pleading with God that we should be given a baby before her. As she agonized over how to tell us her good news, her prayers were answered.

Making rapid changes to Jonathan's pre-Spring Harvest schedule, we agreed to visit the child and his foster mother the next day. Walking down that road must have been one of the most indescribable experiences for both of us. No rounded tummy, hospital visits or ante-natal classes for us. Just a phone call, a walk from the tube station, a ring on the bell of an ordinary terraced house and there was our son. Would we like him? What would we think about him? Would he feel like ours?

In that house which had been a stopping place for hundreds of scraps of humanity, we were ushered into a room where the young daughter of the foster mother was feeding another baby. She went next door and returned with a tiny bundle. The doubts disappeared as we held him, fed him and even changed his nappy. Sarah had been helped a great deal by a very close friend who had recently had a little daughter. She had encouraged her to go and spend as much time with them, bathing and changing the baby and generally experiencing life with a small child so those first few months would not be as terrifying as they could have been.

All too soon it was time to go. How we would have loved to take him there and then.

The Easter weekend was set to complicate Robert's arrival still further, but we were able to persuade the agencies that since we had been helped so much by committed friends, Robert's home was ready and longing for him.

Thursday came, and armed with a shawl made by great grandma and a little suit given by a friend, we drove over to the foster mother's house and made our way home with little Robert.

We are still nervous about the process of letting him know about his background—even though his godfather, Clive Calver, used him as an illustration while preaching at Spring Harvest days after his arrival, of adoption being one of the two ways to become part of a family, and he explains how special it is. (We've got the tape to play to him when he's older!)

Looking back and forward, because we want to start the process again so Robert can have a brother or sister, all we can see is the hand of God, and we're sure that even if God had allowed us to have our own children they could not have been any better than our little Robert.

Useful Address

Care Trust
21a Down Street
London
W1Y 7DN

Tel: 01-499 5949

National Association for the Childless
318 Summer Lane
Birmingham
B19 3RL

[provides infertile couples with advice—
send S.A.E.]

Praying Together

by Mike & Katey Morris

We can all pray on our own. We can know the power of praying with other Christians too.

But what about praying with our marriage partner? Why is it such a problem? Can prayer be fun? Can we worship at home?

If you have ever asked one of these questions, and if you long for greater spiritual unity with your husband or wife, then this book is for you.

This is not a lecture on 'why you should pray more', but a personal and practical manual that will spur you on to action, so that prayer with your partner becomes a living reality, not just some hopeless ideal.

Mike Morris is the Research and Development Officer at the Evangelical Alliance and **Katey** is a secondary school teacher. The seminars that they have led at various Bible-week conventions have shown the enormous need for their practical and spiritual teaching.

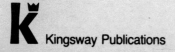

Kingsway Publications